BLOOD SUGAR BLUES

Also by

Miryam Ehrlich Williamson

•

Fibromyalgia: A Comprehensive Approach

The Fibromyalgia Relief Book

BLOOD SUGAR BLUES

OVERCOMING THE HIDDEN DANGERS OF INSULIN RESISTANCE

Miryam Ehrlich Williamson
Foreword by
R. Paul St. Amand, M.D.

Walker & Company
New York

Medical disclaimer: The treatments and therapies described in this book are not intended to replace the services of a trained health professional. Your own physical condition and diagnosis may require specific modifications or precautions. Before undertaking any treatment or therapy, you should consult your physician or health care provider. Special precautions are required for people who are under treatment for Type 1 diabetes. Those with end-stage renal disease should not adopt the dietary changes described in this book. Any application of the ideas, suggestions, and procedures set forth in this book are at the reader's discretion.

First published in the United States of America in 2001 by Walker Publishing Company, Inc.

Published simultaneously in Canada by Fitzhenry and Whiteside, Markham, Ontario L3R 4T8

Library of Congress Cataloging-in-Publication Data
Williamson, Miryam Ehrlich.
    Blood sugar blues : overcoming the hidden dangers of insulin resistance / Miryam Ehrlich Williamson ; foreword by R. Paul St. Amand.
        p.   cm.
    Includes bibliographical references and index.
    ISBN 0-8027-7610-8 (pbk. : alk. paper)
    1. Insulin resistance.   2. Low-carbohydrate diet.   I. Title.

RC662.4.W554 2001
616.3'998—dc21

                                                    2001026347

Printed in the United States of America
4   6   8   10   9   7   5

To Ed, Jeanne, Julie, and Jamie,
whose love nourishes and sustains me

Contents

Foreword

Much of the Western world's population has been assaulted for decades by the less-than-subtle urgings of medical propaganda to avoid fats. Some people have made this a religious endeavor and assiduously complied. But when fat is drastically reduced in the diet, it inevitably is replaced by something else. Often we substitute taste-pleasing carbohydrates.

I wish I had coined the phrase "We live in a society of affluenza." This apt description is an essential part of the explanation for what the American Dietetic Association has called the twin epidemics of diabetes and obesity. But it's not as if we are overindulging in rich foods; quite the contrary may be the case. Some health-conscious people who have cut back on dietary fat while increasing their carbohydrate intake have inadvertently been expanding their waistlines. Worse, those who are susceptible to insulin resistance also have increased their likelihood of developing Type 2 diabetes, as well as heart disease and a variety of other serious health conditions.

This book by Miryam Williamson addresses the problem of insulin resistance—its causes and consequences, and what you can do to slow or reverse this health hazard. A diet high in carbohydrates and sugars is a significant—though not the only—factor in turning insulin into a dysfunctional hormone. When properly nurtured, insulin is a life-sustaining hormone, but as we eat too much starch and sugar, we call upon insulin too frequently, and eventually it may no longer respond appropriately, leading to tissue damage. Simply put, when insulin resistance occurs, it is most often due to the girdle of fat we have amassed.

Carbohydrate ingestion demands the release of insulin. The pancreas responds with a veritable flood of the hormone into the bloodstream. Insulin promotes storage of all the nutritive elements that are not immediately used to meet metabolic needs. It drives protein components—amino acids primarily—into muscles, but also into many other tissues. This hormone also travels to the loading docks of fat cells, where it meets up with circulating lipids. There, it promotes the release of fatty acids from triglycerides. These energy reserves are given an avid reception and begin filling fat cells, our cellular warehouses. Insulin also provides the impetus for the liver to hoard glycogen, strings of glucose held in reserve for future quick release.

Each of these storage facilities sends signals to other tissues, alerting them to the availability of their sequestered nutrients to meet outlying energy demands. The body wastes no food: it stores everything of value, and its zeal to do so makes us fatter. Whatever carbohydrates remain after the gluttonous liver cells have had their fill are readily converted to fat, and three fatty acids are strung into triglycerides, which are transported via the bloodstream throughout the body. The more profound one's insulin resistance is, the more of these energy bundles are generated by the liver, much to the body's detriment.

Overtaxed fat cells eventually begin to resist further expansion of their walls. They join the muscles in a rebellion against the goading of insulin. Tissues simply refuse to accept more fat for storage. However, the pancreas misinterprets this message of noncompliance. It responds by shifting into overdrive and spewing out ever-larger quantities of insulin, as if producing more insulin could actually overcome the mutiny. If tissue resistance progresses, the cells gain a Pyrrhic victory—the cells of the pancreas slowly wither in defeat. Unfortunately, that means the body eventually loses all ability to produce insulin.

When the battle is lost, it usually is because the pancreas has reached its limit of responsiveness to potent and repetitive carbohydrate bombardments. Its maintenance and repair facilities do stretch for a considerable time, but ultimately, as we have seen, they fail to meet the challenge. None of us is endowed with a limitless capacity to produce insulin. The phenomenon of glucose toxicity gradually prevails, although susceptibility to the escalating destruction of insulin-producing cells varies greatly among individuals. But the ultimate fate for many people is a progressive deterioration, beginning with insulin resistance and progressing to diabetes.

The ravages of diabetes are well known to most of us. It impairs circulation, leading to strokes, heart attacks, kidney failure, retinal damage, and the threat of partial or nearly total blindness, progressive disability, and possibly amputations. Yet the threat posed by diabetes to people who are insulin resistant or already diabetic sometimes seems either ill-appreciated or insufficient to sound the alarm. Perhaps false security or an it-won't-happen-to-me attitude keeps people from rigorously making lifestyle changes to safeguard their health. Please heed this warning: destroyed tissues cannot be resurrected! Don't wait too late to change your diet and make the other lifestyle changes outlined in this book.

Insulin resistance must be identified and taken seriously, quite apart from its association with diabetes. At its inception, it may flash not-so-subtle warnings with bouts of hypoglycemia. Such attacks are sufficiently alarming to alert patient and physician alike that all is not working smoothly in the pancreas. Once insulin resistance is in full swing, weight gain progresses—often to fairly massive proportions. A condition that has been named Syndrome X soon follows. It is manifested in blood samples by an abnormal rise in plasma sugar, uric acid, triglycerides, and LDL (bad) cholesterol, and a decrease in HDL (good) cholesterol. Though rarely tested, except in research projects, at this stage insulin remains elevated throughout the day and night. Blood pressure dances up and down, finally refusing to revert to normal.

Miryam Williamson visits this metabolic battlefield. She explores the connection between insulin resistance and autoimmune diseases—including lupus erythematosus, rheumatoid arthritis, and multiple sclerosis; certain cancers; heart disease; high cholesterol and high blood pressure; yeast infections; and various other conditions. Like obesity and diabetes, they are provoked or worsened by the same insulin-resistant metabolic aberrations that lead to chronic hyperinsulinism. Ms. Williamson offers pertinent advice on improving your health and avoiding the ravages of these diseases. For those of you who may be borderline insulin resistant, heeding her words may save you from damage. Her subject is most timely, and though she hardly needs justification or validation, I rush to offer both.

R. Paul St. Amand, M.D.
Assistant Clinical Professor of Medicine
Endocrinology—Harbor/UCLA

Acknowledgments

No book is a solo performance. My name is on the cover of this one, but the book never would have happened without the help and support of dozens of people. I especially thank my husband, Ed Hawes, who saw to it that I was fed while I wrote, assembled and refined the recipes, and served as my first reader; my editor, Jacqueline Johnson, whose foresight, patience, and encouragement meant the world to me; my agent, Jenny Bent, who held my feet to the fire during the proposal-writing stage and made me be better than I am; George Gibson, without whose support this book would not have come into being; and the following people who blessed me with their insight and experience:

Dawn Ahern-Abrams, Michael Anthony, Jan Aplin, Ray Audette, Nancy Ballew, John Brewer, Carole Broderick, Paul Butler, Kate Campion, Treacy Colbert, Jan Cox, Janette Eppler, Steve Feldman, Heather Freed, Cathy Fuller, Kim Garrett, Joe Gedan, Vicki Geis, Richard Geller, Amy Glasband, Eileen Glaser, Richard Geller, Peggy Hartzell, Melissa Henry, Nancy Humeniuk, Jean Johnson, Debby Keen, Nadine Keilholz, Richard Kelly, Christina Loy, Candy Lynch, Diana Mack, Charlotte Merrifield, Janet Mitchell, Lydia Molloy, Todd Moody, Fran Netherton, Ellen Chait Olhsson, Judy Orr, Teresa Parker, Brigitte Poleck, Leanne Ridley, Lee Rodgers, Marra Roscoe, Edward Rosenbluh, Paul St. Amand, Janet Saunders, Randy Shields, Mohur Sidhwa, Dan Smith, Pat Sonnenstuhl, DeAnne Spencer, Brian J. Swinford, Colleen Taylor, Kim Tedrow, Paulette Trumm, Donna Valentino, Joe Valentino, Jay Vercellotti, Patti Vincent, April Willmore, Sandra Winward, Don Wiss, and Craig Wortman.

BLOOD SUGAR BLUES

INTRODUCTION

DESPITE THE BILLIONS of dollars spent on research and development of new medicines and technology for diagnosing and fixing our ailments, our health in the industrialized world is nothing to crow about. True, by the end of the first half of the twentieth century, science had shown us how to survive a host of infectious diseases that used to kill people by the thousands each year. We have vaccines to protect us from influenza, pneumonia, and poliomyelitis. Thanks to antibiotics, a bacterial infection doesn't have to be a death sentence.

However, instead of dying from infection, we die of heart attacks, strokes, and cancers. Chronic diseases such as diabetes are increasing at alarming rates, as is obesity. Too many of us develop autoimmune diseases such as multiple sclerosis and mood disorders such as depression. You might think that this is because, having conquered infection, we have left ourselves open to a host of chronic ailments that were always present but which people used to die too young to contract. In fact, the diseases that plague us today were almost nonexistent in ancient times, and were still rare at the beginning of the twentieth century. Some of them remain unknown to this day in what we like to call "primitive" societies.

There is no disease or disorder that can't be made worse by poor diet. And there is none that can't be improved by changes in lifestyle, especially where nutrition is concerned.

1

This book is about the effect the way we live has on our health and well-being. It is about a dietary mistake that has become almost universal in Western society, and about changes you can make beginning today to reduce or eliminate the symptoms of illness that trouble you. Some 25 percent of the world's population can eat anything they please and never have to think about their weight or the health consequences of their dietary habits. The rest of us need the information this book contains. It is about insulin resistance, a condition in which our cells reject instructions from insulin, the most crucial of our bodies' chemical messengers.

Here you'll learn about the relationship between insulin resistance and the dietary mistake we all make. You'll learn how that mistake causes those of us who are insulin resistant to suffer health problems unknown to our early ancestors—obesity, heart disease, stroke, high blood pressure, arthritis, some types of cancer, diabetes, and more. You'll find guidelines for determining whether you are insulin resistant and, if you are, what you can do about it. You'll learn of various diet plans insulin-resistant people can adopt—not conventional weight-loss diets, but changes in eating habits that you can sustain for a lifetime. You'll be able to compare these plans and decide which suits you best.

As you read this book, you will meet people who have helped themselves to a healthier way of life—people who are successfully dealing with the diseases and disorders associated with insulin resistance. You will read their stories and learn from their experiences. They will inspire you, but even if you know them personally, you will not recognize them here. In order to protect their privacy—and to encourage them to share even the most intimate details of their health and lifestyles—names and other identifying features have been changed. But each of these stories is of a real individual, someone who is happy with what he or she has discovered and eager to help you to a similar success.

Insulin resistance is implicated in a great many diseases and conditions unknown in early times, and still unknown in societies where diets are low in carbohydrates and processed foods are unknown. The list that follows may grow as time goes by and science teaches us more about the action of insulin in insulin-resistant individuals. This is not to say that every disorder on this list is *caused* by insulin resistance, although some are. The relationship between cause and effect is one of the more vexing questions in medicine. Until successive independent studies show beyond doubt that input A is always followed by result B, doctors are reluctant to say that A causes B. This is as it should be. The point here is that some people afflicted with any one of the conditions listed have experienced a reduction in symptoms, if not an outright cure, by changing their lifestyle so as to reduce their bodies' demand for insulin. In the chapters that follow, you will read about the ways in which insulin resistance can cause or contribute to the problems listed here.

CONDITIONS ASSOCIATED
WITH INSULIN RESISTANCE

Autoimmune disorders, including arthritis and multiple sclerosis

Cancer in some forms

Candidiasis (yeast overgrowth)

Celiac disease (sprue)

Chronic fatigue syndrome

Compulsive overeating/food addiction

Depression

Diabetes (Type 2)

Digestive disorders: heartburn, GERD, irritable bowel, inflammatory bowel disease

Gallstones

Gestational diabetes

Heart disease

Hyperlipidemia (abnormal levels of blood fats)
Hypertension (high blood pressure)
Infertility
Obesity
Panic/anxiety attacks
Reactive hypoglycemia
Osteoarthritis
Polycystic ovarian syndrome (PCOS)
Thrombosis (blood-clotting disorder)

That's quite a list, isn't it? For future reference, I suggest you place a mark beside each one that you have experienced. Chances are, if you have checked one, you have checked more than one. If you've felt there was nothing you could do about them, that chronic illness was your fate, you may be in for a pleasant surprise. Diet and lifestyle might not eradicate your condition, but they can make you healthier.

The first step in your quest to control insulin resistance is to accept that your condition is not your fault. Heredity plays a large role in insulin resistance. Second, know that the current low-fat, high-carbohydrate dietary fad is not good for you. Third, while you may never be able to eliminate all tendency to insulin resistance, understand that you can stop it from doing further damage, and in many instances reverse its effects. You can do this without experiencing hunger or feeling deprived. And you will see results in a gratifyingly short period of time.

If you have diabetes and use insulin, you may well benefit from the lifestyle changes discussed in this book. However, because even a slight change in food intake or exercise has implications for the next dose of insulin, I urge you to work closely with your physician.

People with end-stage renal disease who have been instructed to avoid eating proteins must not adopt the way of eating described in this book.

Part I

NUTRITION AND METABOLISM

Experiments have shown that small children who are allowed to choose from an array of healthful, nourishing foods will select those that best meet their nutritional needs. But most people's dietary choices develop along regional and cultural lines, and in recent years food selections have been influenced heavily by government-sanctioned guidelines. Surprisingly, though, for the majority of people the diet promoted by most nutritionists does a poor job of fostering a healthy metabolism and preventing or fighting disease. When it comes to healthful eating, we can learn some valuable lessons by combining the insight of medical science with the instinctive wisdom of our distant ancestors.

·1·
IS WHAT YOU EAT
MAKING YOU SICK?

THE FACT THAT we shop for food instead of collecting it in the wild has a lot to do with the situation in which we find ourselves today. Archaeologists have pieced together a fairly clear picture of the health of our ancestors, the early human beings who date from about 40,000 years ago. Based on their examination of fossil remains, scientists know that these early people were tall and lean, with well-developed, strong bones. There was little or no tooth decay, and barely any evidence of chronic disease. Other indications are that their diet consisted largely of small game animals, birds, reptiles, insects, and eggs. Plant foods—roots, berries, seeds, and nuts—supplied on average no more than 25 percent of an individual's caloric intake, or energy. We can conclude from the condition of archaeological remains that this diet was good for those who ate it.[1]

Cereal grains—the wheat, rye, barley, oats, corn, rice, sorghum, and millet on which most of the world's people today rely for nourishment—were not used as food until much later. There is good reason for this. Cud-chewing animals such as cows and sheep can eat all kinds of vegetation, because they have a second stomach that contains bacteria capable of fermenting fiber. This enables them to extract the nutrients—proteins, carbohy-

1. Nikolas I. Medin, "Food, Health and Homesteading," *Countryside & Small Stock Journal* 83, no. 4, (July/August 1999).

drates, fats, vitamins, and minerals—in plants, twigs, seeds, and grains, getting more energy from their food than they use to digest it.

Human beings cannot digest grains in their natural state. The nutrients in plant foods are enclosed within cells whose walls our stomachs cannot break down. If we eat whole, unprocessed grains, they pass right through our digestive system and show up intact in our feces. To get nutritional use out of grains, we have to grind and cook them. Human beings who lived more than 10,000 years ago couldn't do this, because the first grinding tools were found in the Middle East about 10,000 years ago.[2] It's probably no coincidence that the agricultural revolution, in which people began to domesticate animals and cultivate cereal grains and legumes (peas and beans), started first in the Near East about 10,000 years ago and took some 5,000 years to spread to northern Europe. Without the technology for grinding it, there would have been no reason to grow grain.

The fossil record suggests that a variety of environmental pressures made it necessary to invent a new way of providing nourishment. Large mammals went extinct all over North America, northern Europe, and Asia at approximately the same time that agriculture came into existence. By observing the life cycle of plants in the wild, preagricultural humans may have known how to sow seeds and grow plants long before they started to do so, but as long as game was plentiful and populations were low, there was no motive to engage in farming.

Now, 5,000 or even 10,000 years seems like a long time, but in terms of human evolution it's more like minutes. People who study genetics tell us that the human genome (the entire set of genetic information present in each cell in the body) has undergone little change in the past 40,000 years. In other words, when our ancestors stopped living as hunter-gatherers and turned to agriculture, their bodies failed to adapt to the lifestyle change.

2. Loren Cordain, "Cereal Grains: Humanity's Double-Edged Sword." *World Review of Nutrition and Dietetics* 84 (1999): 19–73.

An abundance of scientific papers argue that wherever diets based on cereal grains replaced the primarily meat-based diet, there was an increase in infant mortality and a shorter life span. Infectious diseases, dental problems, iron-deficiency anemia, and soft bones became more common.

It's interesting to contrast what we know about the diet and physical health of preagricultural hunter-gatherers, who lived more than 10,000 years ago, with the ancient Egyptians of about 5,000 years ago, when agriculture was about 5,000 years old. The Egyptian diet consisted largely of breads, cereals, fresh fruits, vegetables, olive oil, goat milk and cheese, some fish and poultry, and hardly any red meat. The Egyptian diet closely paralleled the one favored today in the Western world, except for refined and processed foods. The techniques for refining sugar and removing the vitamin-rich outer shells of grains did not exist.

Thanks to the Egyptians' custom, over several centuries, of preserving corpses as mummies, scientists have been able to learn a great deal about the health and diseases of ancient Egypt. Many mummies have been found to have overlapping folds of skin, indicating obesity. There is also evidence that dental problems and clogged and scarred arteries were common. Parasites and infectious diseases were widespread. Translations of Egyptian texts of the day describe many of these medical problems. Apparently their diet did not serve them as well as the high-protein, low-carbohydrate diet of the preagricultural human beings, some 5,000 years earlier.

Present-day examples of the effect of lifestyle on human health and appearance are plentiful. The Masai of East Africa are tall and slim people who still live the nomadic life, living mainly on meat and milk from the animals they herd, and picking such greens as they can find in the desert. A few generations ago, the aborigines of Australia and the Maori of New Zealand were just as thin and wiry. Then social and economic forces made them move into the cities and adopt the ways of the dominant society, immigrants from England who displaced them, just as Americans have displaced the indigenous peoples our ancestors found when they came to this continent. Now both the aborigines and Maori are plagued with the same health problems as those whose lifestyle they have adopted.

Closer to home, the Pima Indians on the Gila River Reservation in central Arizona, a half hour south of Phoenix, are a distressing example of what happens to a nation that departs from its ancestral way of life. The Pima Indians have lived in the area for about 8,000 years. They were nearly wiped out by diseases brought to them when the Spaniards came to the desert. Their traditional diet consisted of mesquite, cactus buds, prickly pears, and poverty weeds that grow in the desert. They hunted jackrabbit, mule deer, and white-winged dove. They fished in the Gila River and grew squash and beans in fields irrigated by river water. The nation endured countless cycles of drought and famine. It was a hard existence, but the people survived. In the early 1900s commercial farmers upstream began diverting the Gila River for their own use, leaving the Pima with less and less water. By 1945 Pima Indians were almost entirely unable to live off the land. They began to eat a typical American diet.

There is nothing in historical records to suggest the Pima Indians before 1945 were anything but normally healthy people. In 1963 a research team from the National Institutes of Health descended upon the Pima reservation to study rheumatoid arthritis among the population. They intended to compare this group with the Blackfoot Indians of Montana, to see which group had more people affected by the disease. What they found was that obesity was almost universal among adults, many people weighing more than 400 pounds. The incidence of diabetes was 50 percent. In the general population of the United States, it's a bit over 6 percent. Blindness, circulatory diseases, and kidney failure—serious complications of diabetes—were common. Scientists continue to study the physical makeup of the Pima Indians, but the answer to their physical deterioration seems clear: drastic changes in diet and levels of physical activity have spelled disaster.

It's easy to blame a sedentary lifestyle alone for the prevalence of overweight people, but the role of diet shows up in east-central Africa among the Hutu and Tutsi people of Rwanda and Burundi. A few years ago war between these two nations caught the attention of news media the world over. Because they lived so close to each other, people who heard the news wondered aloud how combatants could tell on sight who was friend and who was foe. The answer is easy. According to Michael Crawford and David Marsh, authors of *Nutrition and Evolution*, the Tutsi, historically, have been the masters and the Hutu their servants. While the Hutu managed the cattle and tended the gardens, meat and milk were reserved for the Tutsi. The Hutu lived on plantains, yams, and other starchy crops. They are short and squat; the Tutsi are tall, lean, and graceful. There is no report of a difference in activity levels between the two groups, but the difference in diet is striking.[3]

Conventional wisdom blames obesity on the consumption of fat, particularly saturated fats found in foods derived from animal sources. But studies of the Inuit nations have shown the opposite. During the long arctic winters they eat nothing but meat, but they remain in good health. It is widely estimated that the typical Inuit diet derives 85 or 90 percent of its total calories from fat, a large percentage of it from saturated fats. Yet chronic diseases are uncommon among the Inuit.

If dietary fat is not the culprit, what is? At least a partial answer may be found in the typical North American diet, which relies so heavily on starchy foods. It wasn't always this way. Until the early 1960s, a proper meal was thought to be centered around proteins. But dietary fashions change, along with the length of skirts and the width of neckties. Gradually in the 1960s and 1970s carbohydrate-rich meals became fashionable. A number of studies blamed heart attacks and strokes on dietary fat. Since fats are associated with proteins more than with vegetables, meat became

3. Michael Crawford and David Marsh, *Nutrition and Evolution*. (New Canaan, Conn.: Keats Publishing, 1995), p. 214.

suspect. Furthermore, many were led to give up meat by concern about Third World poverty, reasoning that more people could be fed per agricultural acre if the land was used to grow carbohydrate-rich grain crops rather than graze protein-providing meat animals.

The low-fat, low-protein, high-carbohydrate trend attracted ever more adherents, reaching its pinnacle in August 1992, when the U.S. Department of Agriculture's Human Nutrition Information Service, acting on the recommendation of the American Dietetic Association, promulgated a new guide to daily food intake. This guide, depicted as a pyramid with carbohydrates at its base, specifies that 55 to 60 percent of calories should be derived from carbohydrate sources, and no more than 30 percent from fats, leaving 20 to 25 percent of caloric intake to proteins. This was a radical departure from the earlier protein-dominant diet that the USDA had endorsed for generations.

In response to the new guidelines, health-conscious Americans altered their diets. Pasta replaced steak as the preferred entree on dining tables and even at banquets across the country. But the new guidelines did not have the desired effect of improving Americans' health. Instead, six years later in October 1998 the American Dietetic Association announced the theme of its eighty-first annual meeting: "The Epidemic of Obesity." Calling it "a public health crisis that affects everyone," the association's news release said, "Obesity contributes to more than 300,000 potentially avoidable deaths each year. . . . Half the population is overweight and a third is obese, according to the latest federal guidelines. Obesity is a major risk factor for a heart attack. Children are affected, as are the elderly and everyone in between."

Still, the American Dietetic Association did not recognize the correlation between an increase in dietary carbohydrates and obesity. What seems to have happened is that after years of a diet that demands large amounts of insulin for energy storage, many people had become immune to their own insulin, the hormone primarily responsible for turning food into energy. This strain on the insulin-producing and -metabolizing mechanisms is of little or no consequence for some people. But for those who are susceptible to insulin resistance—various estimates set our number at between 25 percent and 75 percent of the population—the results are dangerous, and can be devastating.

When you put food into your mouth, you initiate an extensive and complex set of chemical reactions designed to provide you— your brain first, then the rest of your body—with nourishment and energy. Digestion is the mechanical and chemical process of breaking food down into its individual components so they can be absorbed. Metabolism is the transformation of those absorbed substances into materials for providing energy and building new cells. The word *metabolism* comes from a Greek word for "change."

Nutrition science divides the food we eat into three categories, called macronutrients: proteins, carbohydrates, and fats. Proteins are mainly animal products: meat, fish, poultry, eggs, and cheese. Soy is high in protein and may be placed in this category as well. Fats may be saturated, unsaturated, or polyunsaturated (more about this later). Carbohydrate sources include fruits, grains, and vegetables. Some carbohydrates are high in starch, others are not. Fats may be composed entirely of fatty substances, but few proteins or carbohydrates are purely protein or carbohydrate. Meat, fish, poultry, eggs, and cheese all contain fats to a greater or lesser extent, and even some carbohydrate. Carbohydrates may contain proteins and even fats. Nuts are a good example of a composite food. Some nuts are higher in fat and carbohydrate than others, but all three macronutrients are present in all nuts.

Each macronutrient provides some of the many nutrients—vitamins, minerals, amino acids, and fatty acids—necessary to sustain life. The energy they furnish is measured in calories. In an adult whose metabolism is working properly, the amount of energy consumed as food is roughly equal to the amount of energy spent. Such a person neither gains nor loses weight under ordinary conditions. Insulin resistance, as we shall see, is a metabolic malfunction in which the direct relationship between calories in and calories out is disturbed.

Among the macronutrients, proteins break down mainly into amino acids, carbohydrates into sugars, and fats into fatty acids and glycerol. Amino acids assemble themselves to replenish the body's tissues. The average person requires about 300 calories' worth of protein each day—some 70 to 100 grams—to supply the amino acids that the body can't make on its own, and about 75 calories (a bit less than 9 grams) of linoleic acid, the only fatty acid that the body can't make by itself.[4] These are the bare minimum requirements. More calories are needed to provide energy for metabolism and physical activity. It is generally accepted that a person of average size needs about 900 calories a day to sustain life. Proteins and fats contribute to the making of hormones, the chemical messengers responsible for much of what goes on in our bodies. Carbohydrates provide energy, but so do proteins and fats. In fact, carbohydrates perform no function that is not duplicated by proteins and fats. In other words, carbohydrates are not essential to human life.

It is true that carbohydrates turn into glucose, the simple sugar that provides energy to the cells. Glucose is created in plants by a chemical process called photosynthesis that requires sunlight. Plants then convert glucose into a variety of carbohydrates. Animals (human beings included) eat plants to satisfy their need for glucose-derived energy. Human beings require glucose to fuel the brain and red blood cells. Without it we develop hypoglycemia (low blood sugar), an uncomfortable and sometimes dangerous condition (see chapter 4). Glucose is also used in a broad variety of structures in the body, including cell membranes and DNA, the material of heredity. While we must

4. Medin, "Food, Health and Homesteading."

have glucose, we don't need to get it from plant foods. If there's not enough glucose coming from carbohydrates, proteins will make up the deficiency. Even stored fat can provide energy, although not as glucose. The process by which fat becomes energy is known as ketosis. To sum up, while we can live without carbohydrates, we cannot live without proteins and fats.

Starting with the instant when your saliva comes into contact with food in your mouth, the carbohydrates begin to turn into glucose, a simple sugar, which is the energy source your brain and the rest of your body require. How complex the carbohydrate is—that is, how many carbon and oxygen molecules are strung together—plays a dominant role in determining how quickly the resulting glucose will enter your bloodstream. (Table sugar, the result of stripping away the fiber in sugarcane, is a simple carbohydrate. Wheat bran, the outer coating that is removed to produce white flour, is a complex carbohydrate.) Glucose in the bloodstream goes first to the brain, which has first claim on the energy that comes your way. What the brain doesn't need—about 80 percent of most people's total intake—goes to cells that make up the body's organs and muscles. Alerted to the fact that carbohydrates are being digested, your pancreas secretes the hormone insulin.

Insulin has many functions; primarily it pushes glucose out of the blood and into muscle tissue, where it is converted into the energy we need to go about our lives. After a meal or snack, blood sugar levels rise, and insulin does its work. Some glucose gets stored in the liver as glycogen. Typically, the liver stores about a day's worth of glycogen against the time that your body requires an extra energy boost. In times of stress or emergency, hormones from the adrenal glands cause the liver to turn glycogen back into glucose. It is insulin that brings the message to the liver that it's time to release glucose into the bloodstream.

Like all hormones, insulin works by carrying messages from cell to cell. Hormones transmit their information by locking onto receptors on the cells' surface. Receptors function as minute antennae, connected to material called cytoplasm within the cells. In a body that is operating normally, when glucose enters the bloodstream, cells of the pancreas secrete insulin, which connects with insulin receptors on the surface of liver and muscle cells. The insulin receptors instruct the cells to accept glucose and hold onto it until the need arises to spend it for energy.

Four to six hours after a meal, your metabolism shifts gears. Where insulin has been dominant while you digested and metabolized your food, now another hormone comes into play. This is glucagon. It, too, comes from the pancreas. Glucagon suppresses insulin, ensuring that your brain has the glucose it needs but overseeing the shift from carbohydrates to fats as the main fuel for most of the other tissues in the body.

Normally, insulin and glucagon take turns balancing the amount of glucose in your blood, insulin storing it in your liver and muscle cells, and glucagon removing it from storage according to your current need for energy. For this to work properly, though, there must be times when the demand for insulin subsides. Frequent snacks and meals that consist mainly of carbohydrates create an insulin requirement that can overpower the insulin receptors. When this happens, the receptors turn themselves off, the way a highly sensitive electronic device might shut itself down if it received an overwhelming signal in an attempt to protect itself from burning out. The pancreas, lacking the signal that insulin has done its job, responds by releasing even more insulin. The reaction is much like that of a person who has not been heard and therefore speaks in a louder voice.

Insulin resistance occurs when the body's cells stop listening to insulin's instructions. Although the pancreas responds appropriately to the *demand* for insulin production, the body can no longer use its own insulin to convert sugar into energy, nor can it suppress the liver's release of glucose into the bloodstream. At this point there is too much insulin circulating in the blood, try-

HOW INSULIN RESISTANT ARE YOU?

Part 1

1. Do you spend more time than you'd like to worrying about your weight? (Score 1 for yes, 0 for no) _____
2. Do you feel sleepy or fatigued an hour or two after eating? (Score 1 for yes, 0 for no) _____
3. Do you experience anxiety or panic attacks? (Score 1 for yes, 0 for no) _____
4. Score 1 point for every symptom you have from the list below:

    Abnormal triglycerides or cholesterol levels _____
    Binge eating, uncontrollable cravings _____
    Bloating or abdominal gas _____
    Chronic fatigue _____
    Chronic indigestion _____
    Depression that comes and goes _____
    Food/chemical allergies _____
    Gastrointestinal (digestive tract) problems _____
    Heart trouble (heart attack, congestive heart failure, etc.) _____
    Hypertension (high blood pressure) _____
    Inability to lose weight on a low-fat diet _____
    Infertility/irregular menstrual periods _____
    Irritability when hungry _____
    Mental confusion or "brain fog" _____
    Obesity (20 percent or more over your ideal weight) _____
    Panic/anxiety attacks _____

    Total Part 1 _____

Part 2

1. Measure your waist and hips. Divide your waist measurement by your hip measurement.

Women: if the result is .8 or more,
score **10 points** _____

Men: if the result is 1.0 or more,
score **10 points** _____

2. Give yourself 1 point for every blood relative
who has diabetes. _____

3. By how many pounds are you overweight? _____

4. Give yourself 1 point for every time you've gone
on a diet. _____

Total Part 2 _____
Total, Parts 1 and 2 _____

Interpreting the results

Part 1: The maximum possible score is 20. The higher your score, the greater the likelihood that you will benefit from the lifestyle changes outlined in this book.

Part 2: There is no maximum score. If you recorded a 10 in answer to the first question, you are by definition insulin resistant. If you scored the first question as 0 but your total for Part 2 is 15 or more, you have reason to be concerned.

A total for both parts of 35 or more tells you it's time to take action.

ing to knock down the oversupply of glucose. This is hyperinsulinemia, the result of the body's response to excessive insulin production.

When the body can't respond normally to insulin, the hormone is unable to act in its normal fashion on the liver and muscle cells, and so it begins to store excess glucose as fat, both in body tissue and in the blood.[5] Elevated blood fats—cholesterol and trigly-

5. R. A. DeFronzo, "Insulin resistance, hyperinsulinemia, and coronary artery disease: A complex metabolic web." *Journal of Cardiomuscular Pharmacology* 20 (1992): S1-S16.

cerides—are one result. High insulin levels in the blood are also associated with high LDLs (harmful low-density lipoproteins), low HDLs (beneficial high-density lipoproteins), and hypertension.[6] Obesity and heart disease are additional consequences. Excess cholesterol gets stored in a variety of places: in the ovaries as fatty cysts and in the arteries as plaque, for example.

Left unattended, the excessive demand on the pancreas leads to Type 2, non-insulin-dependent diabetes. The good news is that for most people, years may pass before they reach this unfortunate state. One goal of this book is to help people step off the path to Type 2 diabetes. But it's not too late, even if you are already a Type 2 diabetic. The information in this book can help you reduce or eliminate the need for medical intervention.

In some cases, the pancreas gives up and radically reduces or even stops its production of insulin. When this happens, the individual becomes diabetic and must depend on insulin from outside sources, usually by injection. The condition in which the pancreas produces little or no insulin is known as Type 1 diabetes. It usually begins in childhood and has a genetic cause.

> • *EARL: I am a Type 2 diabetic. I know diabetes is supposed to be inherited or caused by obesity, but I don't have any family members who are diabetic, and I'm also not overweight at all. In my opinion, which I have concluded from reading lots of material on diabetes, I wrecked my pancreas, just like lots of Americans are doing. I used to eat tons of carbohydrates a day, and my pancreas would have to respond to this high level of carbohydrate intake. After a period of time, my pancreas just decided it could not produce insulin anymore at the level required to keep my blood sugar levels normal.*
>
> *When I first was diagnosed with diabetes, my doctor put me on an oral agent to help my blood sugar levels return to normal,*

---

6. Shawn P. Kellerman, *The Lifescience Resource* 2, no. 3 (1997).

but because I did not change my diet, the sugar levels continued to be elevated. I was even sent to a registered dietitian to learn how to eat right, but that diet was 60 percent carbohydrates, so that didn't help. The doctor continued to increase my medication until each of the oral meds he tried was maxed out. Then it was time to switch to insulin.

Glucose is a kind of sugar, but it's not the same as the sugar you use to sweeten your coffee. That sugar comes from sugarcane or beets, and you can do quite well without it. Remember that you need an adequate supply of glucose in your blood—and especially in your brain—but this sugar need not come out of the sugar bowl, or even from eating carbohydrates. It's important to keep this distinction straight. The right amount of sugar in your blood keeps you alive, and the sugar in the sugar bowl can contribute to poor heath.

> • CLARICE: *I was fifty when I was diagnosed with Type 2 diabetes. My worst fear came true. One of my earliest memories was hearing that diabetics had to give themselves insulin injections. This horrified me. I've always hated needles. Nobody in my family is diabetic, but I grew up worried that it would happen to me.*
>
> *I was a single mom for many years. I worked as a teacher. When my children finally grew up and left home, I quit teaching and took a good job in high technology so I could work toward a retirement pension. On my first day at work I had to go for an employment physical. When I got back to my office that day, there was a voice-mail message for me telling me to call the company's doctor immediately. My blood sugar was 348—about three times higher than it should have been. I sat at my desk, in shock and in tears.*
>
> *My own doctor reassured me. We'll try diet first, he said, before we talk about needles.*
>
> *That same week, I went to a class on nutrition for diabetics at the local hospital. It was run by a dietitian with the American*

Diabetes Association. When the subject of carbohydrates came up, she told us to follow the standard American nutritional pyramid diet—a little protein and a lot of carbohydrates. My hand went up, and I asked, "Don't unused carbohydrates convert to sugar and store as fat in the body?" The dietitian replied, "All food turns to sugar." That was my last question. I didn't need to hear any more from her.

Before she got her Type 2 diabetes diagnosis, five-foot-four-inch Clarice weighed 180 pounds. Today she's a trim size 12, weighing 140. Her fasting blood sugar is 103. She knows her blood sugar level would soar again if she let up on the lifestyle changes that have led to her success. She knows that her weight problem was a major factor in becoming diabetic, and she's determined not to gain back the weight she's lost.

In the next chapter you'll see that it's not how much we eat, but *what* we eat that brings us to grief.

Part II

DISEASES AND DISORDERS RELATED TO INSULIN RESISTANCE

In one way or another, all of the conditions this book discusses are related to carbohydrate overload and the problems of metabolism that can result. In 1988 Dr. Gerald Reaven, a professor of medicine at Stanford University, pioneered the recognition of the connection among a number of conditions, which he called Syndrome X.[1] A syndrome is a collection of symptoms. This section goes beyond the symptoms of Syndrome X—elevated blood insulin levels, high blood pressure, and high levels of cholesterol and triglycerides in the blood, all of which are risk factors for heart attack—to look at other conditions associated with carbohydrate overload.

1. G. M. Reaven, "Role of Insulin Resistance in Human Disease," *Diabetes* 37 (1998):1595–1607.

·2·
OBESITY

ANIMALS IN THE WILD eat for one reason only: to obtain the energy they need to stay alive. Human beings are different. We eat for energy, to be sure, but we also eat for pleasure. This is why animals in their natural surroundings don't get fat and why, in the simplest of senses, we do. (Actually, animals that sleep through the winter get fat in the fall. But that's fat with a purpose; it keeps them alive while they hibernate. All our fat does is make us feel bulky and unattractive at best, tired and sick at worst.)

Life would be so much easier if recreational eating were the only reason people get fat, but it isn't. I'm sure you know people who can eat like a bear in the autumn and never have to think about their weight. I'm just as sure you know someone—maybe it's you—for whom no amount of dietary restriction gets rid of excess weight and keeps it off. There definitely is more to weight control than just counting calories.

> • RUTH: I'd done enough weight-loss dieting to have lost, and gained back, a few whole people's worth of poundage. At my thinnest I weighed 135 pounds, about 40 pounds too little for my height. At my fattest, well, I stopped getting on the scale when it said 265 pounds, but I didn't start trying to lose weight for another month or more, so I'm not sure where I topped out.

That time I went on an 1,800-calorie diabetic diet. I can thank my genes that I'm not diabetic, but the diabetic diet seemed like something I could follow, and my doctor approved vigorously. I stuck with it for two years and got down to 175 pounds. People said I looked wonderful, but I was feeling awful. I'd cut out sugar almost entirely, I thought. I kept getting more and more tired as the weight came off. Sleepiness overwhelmed me often. I frequently had to pull off to the side of the road and wait for the drugged feeling to pass. I was weak as a kitten, and cranky almost to the point of rage if I happened to get hungry.

I gave up counting calories, resigned myself to the idea that I couldn't weigh what I wanted to weigh. I shifted to a low-fat diet with the emphasis on carbohydrates, the way the U.S. government told me to eat. In five years I gained back 50 pounds. There followed a series of ten-pound losses and gains. I had no more control over my weight than I had over the position of the stars in the sky.

Obesity is a medical term that until recently meant weighing 20 percent above the weight insurance companies have found to be associated with the lowest death rate in a person of a given height. Today the term more often means a condition in which a person is 20 percent to 30 percent over the average weight for his or her age, sex, and height. As such, it is (or should be) a statement of fact, not a value judgment. But doctors are human beings, and most are no less subject than the rest of us to the prejudices that our culture transmits. So it is not uncommon for a doctor to treat an obese person as though he or she were somehow morally inferior, weak-willed, and a glutton. The reality is far more complex, and a doctor with such an attitude is unlikely to help an obese patient find a remedy for the situation.

Obesity is influenced by a variety of factors: heredity, environment, metabolism, and physical activity. Heredity's influence is profound. Some people are simply more prone than others to gaining weight. In a 1990 study at Laval University, Quebec, twelve pairs of identical male twins were fed an extra 1,000 calories a day for three months. They gained between 9 and 29 pounds each. The twins in each pair gained the same amount of weight, but some pairs stored the extra calories as fat while others used them to build muscle.[2]

A University of Pennsylvania study at the same time looked at the weights of nearly 700 pairs of identical and fraternal twins, some of whom had been raised together while others were raised apart. Identical twins have exactly the same genes, having come from a single egg and sperm that split before beginning to develop. Fraternal twins are no more alike in genetic makeup than any other siblings. The idea was to discover how much influence heredity has over obesity. The study found that identical twins, whether raised together or apart, were likely to have similar body weights, while fraternal twins were less likely to weigh the same, whether or not they grew up together. The researchers concluded that the influence of genetic factors is stronger than diet or lifestyle in determining how much a person will weigh.[3]

While it is true that even a modest weight loss can reduce the risk of illnesses associated with obesity—particularly high blood pressure and excessive blood fats—it is also true that some obese people are quite healthy and at no particular risk of obesity-related disease. This suggests that obesity is not a single condition, but rather the result of a complex set of causes with a variety of possible outcomes. It is also possible that any individual case of obesity has more than one cause. And it is obvious that once a person becomes obese, conditions conspire to keep him or her that way.

Some scientists believe overweight people have a genetic makeup that helps them store fat for use in times when food is scarce. This is the so-called thrifty gene theory, first published in

2. C. Bouchard, et al., "The response to long-term overfeeding in identical twins," *New England Journal of Medicine* 322, no. 4 (May 1990): 1477–82.
3. A. J. Stunkard, et al., "The body-mass index of twins who have been reared apart," *New England Journal of Medicine* 322, no. 4 (May 1990):1483–7.

1962.[4] A thrifty gene would help a hunter-gatherer survive when the hunt was going badly, but the advantage turns into a handicap in an environment where three meals a day plus snacks are considered normal. If we never experience times of famine, we simply become insulin resistant and grow fat.

The thrifty gene may be the one that carries the code for an enzyme known as lipoprotein lipase (LPL). This enzyme, produced by fat cells, helps the body to store calories as fat. The more LPL your body produces, the more efficient your body is at storing energy. High LPL levels also make us more likely to regain weight we've lost. A 1990 study at Cedars-Sinai Medical Center, Los Angeles, demonstrated that people who lose large amounts of weight often have higher LPL levels at their new, lower weight than when they began dieting.[5] This is why weight-loss diets don't work. And yo-yo dieting, repeated cycles in which you lose weight and gain back all of it and perhaps even more, can be more harmful than remaining obese. Here's why:

Your body's prime directive is *homeostasis*, which means resisting change. When you start losing weight, your body does everything it can to keep things on an even keel. It doesn't matter that you want to lose weight. Your body reacts to weight loss as if starvation is imminent. It slows down your metabolism—the rate at which you burn glucose for energy—in effect giving you the equivalent of the thrifty gene even if you haven't inherited it. Each time you lose weight and, with the help of the enzyme LPL, gain it back, your regulatory mechanism becomes even more stingy with your energy, making it harder to lose weight the next time. If all you ever do is cut calories, eventually you are likely to start losing lean muscle mass. Muscle burns energy, helping you to lose weight; fat does not. Thus, losing muscle

4. J. Neel, "Diabetes Mellitus: A 'Thrifty' Genotype Rendered Detrimental by 'Progress'?", *American Journal of Human Genetics* 14 (1962):353–362.
5. P. A. Kern, et al., "The Effects of Weight Loss on the Activity and Expression of Adipose-Tissue Lipoprotein Lipase in Very Obese Humans," *New England Journal of Medicine* 322, no. 15 (April 1990): 1053–59.

makes it even harder to lose weight. And on and on it goes. If this cycle sounds painfully familiar to you, don't let discouragement make you give up. In later chapters you will learn what it takes to overcome this tendency. Obesity does not have to be a life sentence.

A combination of psychological and social handicaps often accompanies obesity. Discrimination against obese individuals is widespread in industry and the academic world. Studies have shown that obese people are more likely to be denied employment or promotion. They are often assumed to be lazy or to lack willpower. As is true with oppressed minorities, obese people tend to adopt these judgments themselves, feeling guilty, becoming depressed, and lacking a sense of self-confidence or self-worth. These feelings are often associated with decreased activity of the brain chemical serotonin. Unfortunately, serotonin deficiency can cause depression, and often gives rise to cravings for the raw material that creates serotonin—the amino acid tryptophan, plentiful in starches and sweets. These cravings can seem almost irresistible, causing more weight gain and giving the cycle another spin.

There is probably some good evolutionary reason why we were born to love the taste of sweetness. You need only feed a baby alternate spoonfuls of pureed squash and applesauce to be convinced that the preference for sweetness is inborn. In some of us, though, it becomes an addiction that is difficult—but not impossible—to overcome.

For some people the craving is restricted to one sort of food—chocolate or doughnuts, for example. Some people crave bread, the whiter and doughier the better. It's fairly common for someone trying to beat a craving for sweets to shift to bread or bagels on the theory that at least those are real foods. Physiologically, there's not much difference between what happens when you eat a sweet and when you eat white bread. Both begin to turn into sugar as soon as they come into contact with the saliva in your mouth and enter the bloodstream almost instantly.

Cravings can rule your life. Ask any recovering alcoholic about that. If you've ever attended an Alcoholics Anonymous meeting, you probably noticed the way many members consumed sweets. Alcoholic drinks are made from grain or fruit, both rich sources of sugar. Addiction to carbohydrates is quite different from being addicted to alcohol, but both begin as an effort to blunt pain, whether physical or psychological, by increasing the feel-good chemicals in the brain.

> • *GINGER: I'm a Type 2 diabetic on insulin. I weighed more than 400 pounds for the past ten years. Right now I'm down to 380, but lately I've let myself eat some of the things I never should touch, and I'm gaining again. I can remember as a teen craving comfort foods and then getting into a stupor after I ate them. I used food as a pacifier instead of dating or having fun. I've never tried heroin, but I know what a heroin addict feels like. I'm like that with food.*
>
> *When you're addicted to food, the urge to eat grows stronger, and the feeling of satisfaction after you eat lasts for shorter and shorter periods of time, until you get so out of control that you're spending your whole day thinking about what you're going to eat. You know that every time you put something into your mouth you're making your health problems worse, but you need to eat more and more. You just keep spiraling down.*
>
> *Everyone knows I'm on this downward spiral. It makes me want to curl up and hide. But still there's that hold that food has over me. In spite of the feeling of panic I have knowing I'm shortening my life, at the same time there's the comfort that food gives me.*
>
> *I know I've got to get my eating under control. It's amazing how many excuses I can come up with to keep from doing it one more day.*

After a while on a low-carbohydrate diet, you will be free of food cravings. How long that will take depends on the severity of your addiction. If you're determined to fend off addictive behavior but aren't quite ready for a major change in your way of eating, here are some things you can do.

> • *EVAN: By the time I was thirty-five, I weighed about 265. I'm six-foot-two inches tall, so I could get away with a lot, but this was too much. I kept talking about losing weight. My problem with overweight had to do with male-female relationships. I think there's a natural problem there. If a person is a lot overweight, they're less likely to have a good relationship with a significant other.*
>
> *I'm an addictions counselor. A long time ago I examined the tenets of the Overeaters Anonymous program. I knew that one of the things you do in Alcoholics Anonymous is admit you are powerless over alcohol. I understand that alcoholism is a biochemical reaction, and I discovered that the OA people say you need to identify the food groups that you can't eat and accept that they are the ones you're powerless over. That dovetails nicely with low-carbohydrate eating. I'm powerless over high-carbohydrate foods.*
>
> *I found the more I stayed away from carbohydrates, the easier it was to stay away. Especially in the first weeks, it's very important for you to have plenty of whatever high-protein foods you enjoy around to eat: cheeses, meats, things like that. Instead of thinking of all the foods you can't eat, make a shopping list of the high-protein, high-fat things you can eat and stock up so there will always be something around that you can eat when you feel like eating.*

First, try to be rigorously honest in distinguishing between real physical hunger and mouth hunger, the desire to eat when you don't really need to. Do you get hungry an hour or two after a meal? If you think of eating before your stomach has fully emptied, it's a good bet that you've just had a drop in blood sugar caused by insulin resistance, and that the carbohydrates in your last meal caused it.

Cravings are a step beyond hunger, though. Craving takes over your consciousness. A real craving won't leave your mind alone until you satisfy it. Preferably while you're not craving anything, think about the situations that trigger cravings. Do you find yourself obsessing about a particular food or about eating in general? Is the obsession triggered by anything in particular—an emotionally charged event? Some kind of personal interaction? A visual cue such as a photo of something that looks good to eat? If so, is there some way you can avoid that particular stimulus? Some way you can defuse it if you can't avoid it? Often, if you give it a few minutes' thought, you can find a way to prevent this particular trigger in the future. You may find that if you merely delay eating for the time it takes to consider the stimulus and what to do about it, the craving is gone for a while, or at least less urgent and more manageable.

• *MIRYAM: My big triumph came about six months into my new low-carb way of eating. I had to attend a banquet at a conference where I was one of the speakers, so there was no way to get out of it. It was a buffet, which isn't a good idea for someone with an eating problem. There were several stations, all with various kinds of ethnic foods. I've got to admit I was pretty anxious about finding food that was okay for me.*

It turned out fine. Every station had some kind of protein dish that wasn't breaded or drenched in gravy. The last station was the dessert table. I skipped it, with regret. After I'd finished eating, I decided I'd been so good for six months that I could give myself permission to have dessert. I thought about it long and hard, and then went to the dessert station and picked up a plate. Everything had chocolate in it or on it. I was a nut for chocolate six months before. I looked at each item and thought about whether I really wanted it. I must have stood there for five minutes thinking, "No, that will be too sweet. Uh-uh, too rich," and finally I put down the plate and went back to my seat. I really, honestly, didn't want dessert. That was the first time in my life that I had the opportunity to indulge in all the chocolate I could eat, and turned it down.

Sometimes we perceive hunger when what we're really experiencing is thirst. Many people find it helps to take a big drink of water when a craving hits. Again, there is the element of delay in satisfying the craving that may make it go away. If the cause of the hungry feeling is acid reflux, a backup of digestive juices where they don't belong, drinking water may relieve the hungry feeling. Just satisfying the thirst may relieve the craving, or make it less urgent and more manageable. Try to wait fifteen or twenty minutes before deciding whether the water helped.

While you're waiting for the water to get into your cells and stop your thirst, try a change of environment. Go for a short walk outdoors, if that's possible, or down the hall if you're at work. If you can't go anywhere else, go to the bathroom, wash your hands and face, and go back to where you were.

If by then you're still thinking about eating something in particular, will a substitute help? Eating a sugary treat guarantees that the craving will come back again soon. Perhaps something that is largely protein will help—a hard-boiled egg, a piece of cheese, or a stalk of celery stuffed with cream cheese and olives or peanut butter (or, even better, almond butter; many peanut butters contain added sugar) are good choices that support the low-carbohydrate, high-protein way of eating.

If all else fails—and I know this is going to horrify some people—give in to your craving, but do it in style. Give your full attention to what you're doing while you feed yourself the food you crave most. Set a place at the table, or move things away on your desk and set yourself up there, using a napkin for a place mat. Put all the food you think you want out in front of you. Use utensils, rather than eating with your fingers. Make an event of it. If you're where you can, play background music. Don't read.

Pay attention to what you're eating. Get all the pleasure out of it that you possibly can. Treat yourself as you would treat a dear friend who deserved a feast.

If you start feeling guilty, try to refocus your thoughts on the pleasure of eating. If you start feeling as though you've had enough, promise yourself the food will be available to you later if you want it, and store away what remains. The important thing is not to punish yourself by overeating, or for overeating. It is reasonable to hope for the day to come when you are able to change this behavior. A change of diet will help make this possible. Meanwhile, until that day comes, don't make things worse by refusing to let yourself enjoy what you eat.

If you are obese as a result of out-of-control cravings, you should consider getting extra support while you change your lifestyle. Appropriate dietary changes described in this book are very likely to eliminate your cravings and cause you to lose weight. However, if there are also psychological reasons that cause you to overeat, they will probably not go away without help. Also, beware of the tendency to replace one addiction with another.

·3·
HEART DISEASE, HIGH BLOOD PRESSURE, AND HIGH BLOOD FATS

ULTIMATELY ALL creatures die, even those that are perfectly healthy. The body's cells divide and divide again as part of the process of life. If they follow the pattern built into them, dividing cells simply form new tissue identical to that which is wearing out and needs to be replaced. If they deviate from the built-in pattern, dividing cells become cancer. But sooner or later, no matter how faithfully they have adhered to the pattern, there will come a time when the cells have done all the dividing they can do, and the individual slips into death. That's how it is for people who have managed to avoid the viral and bacterial infections, pollution and toxins, accidents and injuries, and diseases of civilization that shorten the lives of most people: a gradual diminution of the cells' ability to divide and replace outworn tissue, a gradual descent into death—no pain, no suffering, just a quiet letting go.

That's how it should be for all of us, but it happens so rarely that you may never have known anyone who died that way. But if you have, you may have learned not to fear death. And you may have made up your mind that's the way you want to die. And that may be why you are reading this book.

As it is, few people in Western society die of plain old age. To my way of thinking, death from any cause other than plain wearing out is a premature death. Heart disease is the leading cause of premature death. Cerebrovascular stroke, the third most common cause, is discussed in this chapter because some of the same mechanisms that cause heart attack can just as easily cause stroke. Cancer, the second most common cause of early death, is dealt with later.

The links between heart attack and high blood pressure are well known. So are the links between cerebrovascular stroke and high blood pressure, and obesity and high blood pressure. Somewhat less well known are the connections among hyperlipidemia (high levels of cholesterol and some forms of fat in the blood), blood clots, and heart attack and stroke. Hypertension, hyperlipidemia, and the tendency to blood clots are so closely related that most people who have one of these have one or both of the others. Yet it happens far too often that a doctor will prescribe two or three different medicines to treat them, as though there were no relation among them. A more realistic approach is to see each of these conditions as a symptom of an underlying disease—insulin resistance.

In this, the failure to recognize insulin resistance as a disease entity in its own right and start the treatment there stems from the reluctance of many physicians to recognize that one can be insulin resistant without being diabetic, let alone that something as serious and common as insulin resistance can be brought under control by modest lifestyle changes. Yet that is a fact.

HYPERTENSION

The common belief, among both health care professionals and the general public, is that obesity and eating too much salt are the causes of high blood pressure. It is true that sodium (the main ingredient in table salt) causes fluid retention, and that excess fluid in the cells is associated with high blood pressure. It is probably true that people who have high blood pressure should avoid salt as much as possible. Many overweight people have high blood pressure, just as many who have high blood pressure are obese. It has been shown that even a small weight loss brings about a slight lowering of blood pressure. But blaming overweight and salt intake for high blood pressure overlooks the abundance of clinical studies that have found an unusually high number of people with hypertension who are also insulin resistant.

• *JIM: I was a pretty healthy guy until I started having trouble sleeping. I had always been a light sleeper, but suddenly I found myself waking up at every little noise. My wife and I had to stop sleeping together because I would wake up every time she moved in bed, and then I wouldn't be able to get back to sleep. I became a vegetarian, because I heard it would help my body work better and reduce stress. Then one New Year's Eve we had a party. I couldn't really enjoy myself because I felt like I was getting sick. Sure enough, the next day I came down with a very bad cold. I usually get over colds very fast, but this one lingered and lingered, and the longer it lasted, the worse my sleep got, until I wasn't sleeping at all most nights.*

In February my wife made me go to the doctor. The doctor didn't do anything for my cold and ignored my sleep problem, but she expressed concern with my blood pressure. It was about 165 over 100. She put me on blood pressure medication, which she said would help the insomnia. It didn't. She tried a whole slew of medications: beta blockers, and something with calcium, and a whole bunch of other stuff. I can't remember all of them. None of them worked at all. It didn't matter what medication or how much I took, my blood pressure stayed high. Then she began prescribing medication for the sleep problem, thinking that maybe if I could sleep better, my blood pressure would come down. None of them worked.

Between one-quarter and one-third of lean people with high blood pressure are insulin resistant.[1] And even thin people with

1. Gerald M. Reaven and Ami Laws, eds., *Insulin Resistance: The Metabolic Syndrome X* (Totowa, N.J.: Humana Press, 1999), p. 286.

hypertensive parents but normal blood pressures show high blood insulin levels (hyperinsulinemia), indicating insulin resistance. Lowering insulin levels in the blood results in lower blood pressure, while lowering blood pressure does not result in lower blood insulin levels. Dr. Lewis Landsberg, dean of the Northwestern University Medical School, says insulin resistance and hyperinsulinemia raise blood pressure, which may be an important cause of hypertension in patients for whom no other reason can be identified.[2]

Health-related articles often refer to hypertension as a silent killer. Although symptoms may include a throbbing headache on awakening that disappears when you are up and about, dizziness, increased muscle tension, blurred vision, nausea, and vomiting, most people who have high blood pressure experience no symptoms at all. Blood pressure can soar to extremely dangerous levels before any symptoms appear. The only way to detect high blood pressure is to have a reading taken periodically.

Other factors, including kidney disease, an overactive thyroid gland, and a tumor on the adrenal glands, may also cause hypertension, which may explain why some people have high blood pressure but not high insulin levels. No evidence has been found to blame insulin resistance for gland-related hypertension.

Health care professionals are familiar with what they call white coat hypertension, in which the patient's blood pressure readings are elevated because of the anxiety associated with a visit to the doctor's office. According to Dr. Ken Grauer, about 20 percent of patients diagnosed with hypertension have high readings only in the doctor's office.[3] For this reason, it is often a good idea to have your blood pressure measured several times in different

2. L. Landsberg, "Insulin Sensitivity in the Pathogenesis of Hypertension and Hypertensive Complications," *Clinical and Experimental Hypertension* 18, nos. 3–4 (1996): 337–46.
3. Ken Grauer, M.D, "Management of Hypertension: JNC-VI Guidelines and Beyond," Online Coverage of the 50th Annual Meeting of the American Academy of Family Physicians Scientific Assembly, September 16–20, 1998; http://www.medscape.com.

locations and under different circumstances before arriving at a diagnosis of hypertension.

> • JIM: *My wife switched from being a vegetarian to low-carbohydrate eating in hopes that it would help her overcome fatigue and rheumatoid arthritis. I didn't approve, but I kept my mouth shut. Two days after she started eating that way, she didn't need an afternoon nap and she started looking healthier, so I decided to try it, too.*
>
> *After a week my blood pressure came down a couple of points. It wasn't much, but it was the first time it had come down at all. Then, after three weeks it really began dropping. I went from the 160s over 100s to the 140s over low 90s practically overnight. Then the next week I started getting consistent readings of about 130 over 80 and sometimes even lower. This was where I was supposed to be. This was so amazing. I had tried virtually every single blood pressure drug on the market, and not one of them had done a thing for me. Now eating meat and almost eliminating carbohydrates had accomplished what the doctors had been unable to do.*

While the link between insulin resistance and high blood pressure is clear, the exact mechanism by which excessive blood insulin operates in hypertension is less clear. There are several possibilities, based on what we know about the actions of insulin. It is possible they may all be correct. One theory starts with the fact that insulin arouses the sympathetic nervous system, the part of the nervous system that is not under your conscious control. When blood insulin levels are chronically high, the sympathetic nervous system is working all the time. One of the effects of sympathetic nervous system stimulation is the release of norepinephrine, one of the adrenal stress hormones. Norepinephrine can be detected in the urine when the sympathetic nervous system is stimulated. High levels of urinary norepinephrine and insulin have been found to be related both to each other and to hyper-

tension. When insulin is suppressed, however, both norepinephrine levels and blood pressure decrease.[4]

You might guess from this that sympathetic nervous system
stimulation is the cause of both insulin resistance and hypertension rather than the reverse. But studies of hypertension associated with obesity show that insulin resistance begins before
blood pressure starts to rise. This is more evidence of the primary
role of insulin resistance in high blood pressure.

Another possible mechanism stems from the fact that high levels of insulin correlate with low levels of sodium in the urine. Insulin causes the kidneys to retain sodium and keep it from being
secreted in urine, allowing it to return instead to the bloodstream. Homeostasis, in this case an effort to keep the blood
from getting too salty, leads to an increase in the amount of water in both the bloodstream and the rest of the body's cells. Water retention makes it harder for blood to flow through the
circulatory system, because of the added pressure that swollen
tissues exert on arteries and veins.

Insulin also increases blood pressure by making artery walls
less elastic and altering the mechanical action of the blood vessels. Insulin acts like growth hormone on smooth muscle cells in
the arterial walls. Increased insulin levels stimulate the smooth
muscle cells and make them larger. As they grow, they make the
arterial walls thicker, stiffer, and less supple. This decreases the
volume of blood within the arteries, forcing the heart to exert
more pressure to force the blood through these narrowed, more
rigid arteries.[5]

Blood pressure measurement gauges the pressure on the walls
of blood vessels as the heart pumps blood through the body.
Two measurements are taken, and the result is expressed in mil-
limeters of mercury (mm Hg) as a fraction. The upper number
signifies systolic pressure, the force exerted when heart muscle

4. Landsberg, "Insulin Sensitivity."
5. Michael R. Eades and Mary Dan Eades, *Protein Power* (New York: Bantam
Books, 1996), p. 317.

fibers shorten and the heart contracts; the lower number is diastolic pressure, the reading when heart muscle is exerting the
least amount of pressure. Systolic pressure indicates how elastic
the blood vessels are. Diastolic pressure gives an idea of how
clogged the blood vessels are.

There are two common misconceptions about blood pressure
readings. One is that the systolic number is not important as
long as the diastolic number is acceptable. The other is that a systolic number that equals 100 plus your age is normal. Neither is
correct. In 1987 the Framingham Heart Study identified high
blood pressure in general and high systolic pressure in particular
as a significant predictor of sudden death.[6]

Current thought is that, at any age, a systolic reading that is
consistently above 130 or a diastolic reading above 85 is too high.
Malignant hypertension—a reading above 160/100—brings the
risk of severe damage to blood vessels. Left unchecked, malignant
hypertension is likely to result in death.

Congestive heart failure (CHF) can occur if hypertension goes
untreated for too long. The term is a bit inaccurate, since it im-
plies that the heart has stopped working, which is not the case.
CHF is a condition in which the heart has weakened and is no
longer up to the task of moving an adequate supply of blood to
the body's organs and tissues. Causes include damaged heart
muscles and faulty valves. When blood backs up in the heart,
fluid collects in surrounding tissues, including the lungs and
liver. Symptoms of heart failure include shortness of breath even
at rest, especially when lying down, and edema (fluid retention)
throughout the body. Often, severely swollen legs and feet are an
early sign of congestive heart failure.

• *KAY: I used to consider myself healthy, even though I've always
been overweight. I've lost 100 pounds at least three times, but my*

6. B. E. Kreger, A. Cupples, and W. B. Kannel, "The Electrocardiogram in Pre-
diction of Sudden Death: Framingham Study Experience." *American Heart
Journal* 113 (1987):377–382.

blood pressure remained normal, even though there is hypertension throughout my family. My weight never kept me from doing anything I wanted to do.

Four years ago I found myself in circumstances that were very difficult emotionally, and I completely lost control of my weight. By the time I reached 400 pounds, it was getting very hard to walk. I was out of breath all the time. Even talking was difficult; I'd get to breathing so hard I'd have to stop and wait to catch my breath. It got so bad that I'd have to drive my children to the store, give them a list, and tell them to go in to do the shopping.

I was carrying a lot of weight in my abdomen and stomach. I later learned most of it was water from congestive heart failure. It made my stomach hard as a wall. Any pressure hurt. There were times during sex that my heart felt like it was going to explode. It was really scary.

My doctor sent me to a cardiologist. The cardiologist told me he had seen people who weighed more than 600 pounds and didn't have as much trouble with their hearts, but that my weight was making it too hard for my heart to function. He told me, "If you don't lose weight, you have maybe five years left to live." I was forty-six, and scared out of my wits. I told him about all the yo-yo dieting I'd done, how I could lose 100 pounds and gain back 120. The doctor said, "Then the only thing we can do for you is a gastric bypass." He referred me to a surgeon.

That doctor had a year-long waiting list, but because of my situation his office got me an appointment in six months. While I was waiting, I saw a dietitian who put me on a low-fat diet. I lost about twenty pounds while I waited for my surgical appointment.

The surgeon explained the gastric bypass. They make the food go around your stomach. There's a small pouch below the stomach that can only hold three ounces of food. His nurse showed a video that told how I was going to have to eat after the bypass: three little meals a day—an ounce each of meat, potato, and a vegetable. They put a band around the pouch to keep anything larger from

going through into your intestine. If you eat more than you're al-
lowed, you just throw it back up. It's like an enforced fast, except
that you're not supposed to feel hunger because your stomach is
out of the loop, so to speak.

For the rest of your life you have to take vitamins because
you're getting so little food, and you're not absorbing nutrients
very well, anyway. They scheduled me for the operation two
months from the time of my appointment. That gave me time to
think and pray for another solution.

HIGH CHOLESTEROL

Another symptom of insulin resistance commonly treated as a
disease in its own right is the overabundance in the blood of cholesterol and harmful blood fats. Cholesterol is a waxy substance
made mainly in the liver, but if the liver can't make as much as
your body needs, then other parts of your body leap into action.
The amount of cholesterol in your blood has little to do with the
amount of cholesterol in your diet. The average American con-
sumes between 300 and 450 milligrams of cholesterol a day,
while the body makes 800 to 1,500 milligrams. An enzyme
called HMG CoA reductase controls the manufacture of cholesterol in the liver. This is the enzyme that is blocked by the so-
called statin drugs prescribed to lower serum cholesterol. But
the body has its own way to control HMG CoA reductase: the
hormones insulin and glucagon. Insulin stimulates the enzyme,
causing the liver to turn out more cholesterol. Glucagon has the
opposite effect, causing your liver to manufacture less cholesterol. Reducing the body's demand for insulin is a drug-free way
to control high cholesterol.

Cholesterol is measured in milligrams (mg) per tenth of a liter
(deciliter, or dl; a liter is a bit more than a quart). People concerned about preventing heart attacks tend to become fixated on
their cholesterol level as the number of primary importance.
Conventional wisdom says that you should worry if your cholesterol count rises above 200 mg/dl; some say that people under

thirty should keep their level below 180. It's easy to infer from this that the lower your cholesterol level, the better off you are. In fact, there is no convincing evidence linking a high cholesterol reading alone with illness or death. According to Dr. Joseph Risser, director of clinical research at Lindora Medical Clinics, the death rate rises in people whose numbers are below 160, and having a cholesterol reading below 140 is at least as dangerous as having one above 240.

The blood fats consist of lipoproteins and triglycerides. Their levels are also reported in a blood cholesterol test. Low-density lipoproteins (LDLs) are the "bad" ones, although they're not entirely bad. They carry cholesterol to the tissues. You want their number to be low, but not too low, since you need that cholesterol to keep your cells intact and to help in the manufacture of hormones. The generally accepted healthy range for LDLs is 130 to 160. High levels of LDLs are associated with increased risk of heart disease.

High-density lipoproteins (HDLs) are the "good" ones. They carry excess cholesterol from the tissues to the liver, where the cholesterol is processed and sent to the bile for elimination. The desirable range for HDLs is 55 to 150. HDLs are believed to lower your risk of heart disease. Recently, scientists have begun to break down lipoproteins into very-low-density lipoprotein (VLDL) and intermediate-density lipoprotein (IDL.) When it comes to lipoproteins, the lower the density, the higher the risk of heart attack.

The most important numbers in your serum cholesterol test are triglycerides and HDLs. If you divide your total cholesterol count by the number for HDLs, you get your cardiac risk factor. The higher the result is, the higher the statistical risk that you will develop a heart condition. A risk factor below 4.44 is desirable.

Triglycerides are fats in your blood that are not associated with proteins. They are made in the liver from glycerol, which is the carbohydrate part of fat, and fatty acids. As is true for cho-

lesterol, you can't get along without triglycerides. While cholesterol is used in part to build and maintain the body's structure,
triglycerides provide energy. They hitch a ride on the lipoproteins and travel to the cells, where they are burned for energy or
stored for future use. The recommended range for triglycerides
is 30 to 160. Ideally, you will keep them below 100. By now you
can probably guess what is to blame if your triglycerides are too
high: overproduction of insulin, the result of insulin resistance.

There is no evidence of any connection between how much fat
you eat and your risk of heart disease. One survey by the U.S.
government involving 4,700 people failed to find any evidence
of risk associated with elevated total cholesterol regardless of age
or sex.[7] And a recent study finds that once people get into their
late eighties, the higher their cholesterol reading, the longer they
are likely to remain alive.[8]

If cholesterol and triglycerides simply kept floating around in
your bloodstream, they probably wouldn't do much harm and
would be no cause for concern. Unfortunately, that's not how it
works. Excess blood fats can build up in the blood and accumulate in the walls of the blood vessels. These deposits are called
plaques; the condition they cause is known as atherosclerosis.
The term describes a situation in which fatty buildup narrows the
passageway through which blood can flow, depriving portions of
the heart, brain, or lower limbs of blood. Apparently, cholesterol
alone does not do this; triglycerides must be overabundant as
well.

The third factor that contributes to the development of heart
disease is excessive clotting of the blood. Like so many processes
that our bodies undertake, clotting is a two-edged sword. When
you are injured in a way that causes bleeding, either externally or
internally, you want a clot to form as quickly as possible. Where

7. Richard K. Bernstein, M.D., *Dr. Bernstein's Diabetes Solution* (Boston: Little,
Brown, 1997), p. 260.
8. J. Raloff, "High Cholesterol May Benefit Elderly," *Science News* 152, no. 17
(October 25, 1997): 260.

tissue is damaged, a blood clot is like the lid on a bottle. It keeps the contents from flowing out of its container. The hereditary disease in which the ability to clot is missing is called hemophilia. It is a life-threatening condition.

If you've ever donated blood, you know that losing as little as a pint can leave you feeling a bit weak, light-headed, and short of breath. A pint of blood is a small portion of the five or six quarts that make up your total blood supply, yet you notice the decrease in blood volume. Those feelings quickly disappear if you drink plenty of fluids and eat a good meal. Under normal circumstances your body's impulse toward homeostasis makes it good at making new blood cells to replace those you've given away. Nevertheless, losing blood is a serious matter. Your body depends on a certain volume of blood flowing through your arteries and veins to carry glucose and oxygen to your tissues and, in particular, to your brain, your entire being's first priority. Clotting aids homeostasis by minimizing the amount of blood you lose when you are injured.

But an excessively strong tendency toward clotting can be as dangerous as the failure to clot. In the course of normal life, tiny blood clots form and dissolve in the bloodstream with frequency. Clotting is handled by a substance called tissue plasminogen activator (t-PA). Its action is balanced by plasminogen activator inhibitor-1 (PAI-1). PAI-1 is increased by insulin. The level of PAI-1 in the blood is directly related to obesity, LDLs, triglyceride levels, and hypertension. The omentum, an organ in the belly made up of fat cells and connective tissue, manufactures PAI-1.[9] The bigger the omentum, the more PAI-1 is produced, and the more likely blood is to clot. Narrow blood vessels make blood move more slowly, increasing the tendency to clot. Plaques on blood vessel walls sometimes rupture, giving rise to clotting if the balance between t-PA (the substance that moderates clotting) and PAI-1 (which prevents t-PA from doing its

9. Reaven and Laws, *Insulin Resistance*, p. 324.

job) is favorable to clotting. So we have a situation in which people who are insulin resistant have a greater than normal tendency to develop blood clots. The formation of a blood clot in an artery or vein is a life-threatening event, made even more dangerous when the passage of blood is already slowed by thickened and hardened blood vessel walls.

Three factors, then—all closely interrelated—favor the development of heart disease and heart attacks. These are hypertension, fatty buildup on blood vessel walls, and the formation of blood clots. To make things even more circular, damaged fatty plaque on blood vessel walls can cause blood clots to form, and clots can damage blood vessel walls. And behind it all is insulin gone wrong.

·4·
Glucose Intolerance and Hypoglycemia

GLUCOSE INTOLERANCE describes a situation in which blood glucose levels are higher than they should be, but not high enough to warrant the diagnosis of diabetes. Impaired glucose tolerance by itself produces no symptoms, although it may be accompanied by other problems such as obesity. Higher-than-normal blood sugar doesn't necessarily cause the serious complications associated with diabetes. However, about 25 percent of people with impaired glucose tolerance go on to develop Type 2 diabetes.

If you have a routine physical examination every year or two, as you should, you will probably be sent to the laboratory before breakfast to have blood drawn. Your blood sample will undergo several tests. One will be a fasting blood sugar test, which determines how much glucose is present when you haven't eaten for the past eight hours or more. Some doctors look for sugar in a urine sample, but many consider this inadequate to rule diabetes in or out.

Most doctors consider a fasting blood glucose of 126 or more to indicate diabetes. Some are reluctant to render the diagnosis on the basis of one test alone and may ask for one or two additional fasting blood glucose tests, or a nonfasting test done once or twice. For postprandial testing, a blood sugar measurement of 200 or higher is considered to indicate diabetes. A fasting glucose between 115 and 125 is suspicious and warrants followup testing after a few months have gone by. Some doctors, seeing a fasting glucose this high, will order an oral glucose tolerance test, in which you are asked to drink a solution containing either 50 or 100 grams of glucose. Blood is then drawn every half hour to an hour for two to five hours. People whose blood sugar shoots up rapidly and comes down slowly are termed hyperglycemic (hyper = too much) and may be headed for diabetes. Those whose blood sugar spikes and then drops suddenly—this may not happen until the third or fourth hour, which is why a five-hour test is preferable—are reactive hypoglycemics (hypo = too little). Patients showing either of these results are said to have impaired glucose tolerance.

Some doctors also order a test called hemoglobin Alc. This measures the average number of sugar molecules attached to red blood cells. Some also recommend a fasting insulin test, but there is less agreement about the accuracy and usefulness of this test.

Certain factors can interfere with glucose tolerance and give an erroneous reading. These include having eaten fewer than 150 grams of carbohydrate a day for three days before the test, having spent the last few days in bed, or having been physically inactive for the last few weeks.[1] Extreme physical stress, certain drugs (diuretics, beta blockers, and steroids), smoking during the test, and anxiety over needle sticks can yield a false result indicating impaired glucose tolerance.

Hypoglycemia might appear to be the opposite of diabetes, but diabetics can experience hypoglycemia, too. Insulin-dependent diabetics can become hypoglycemic if they inject more insulin than they need, if they wait too long to eat after injecting insulin, or if they engage in unaccustomed exercise. Diabetic hypoglycemia is dangerous. In a person who takes insulin, it can result in loss of consciousness, convulsions, and even death. Things don't often get that dramatic in a person who doesn't have dia-

1. *Cecil Textbook of Medicine*, 20th ed. (Philadelphia: W. B. Saunders, 1996), p. 1259.

betes, but hypoglycemia can still be dangerous, especially if you drive or work around machines.

Normally, when insulin sends blood sugar levels too low, adrenaline brings it back up, and the healthy individual is largely unaware of the changing concentration of glucose in the blood. However, if you are insulin resistant, you are apt to develop *reactive* hypoglycemia—a drop in blood glucose that can happen gradually over two or three hours after a meal, or suddenly and dramatically. Another term for reactive hypoglycemia is postprandial (after-meal) hypoglycemia.

SYMPTOMS OF HYPOGLYCEMIA

Feeling sleepy to the point of feeling drugged

Mental confusion, inability to concentrate,
   impaired memory

Dizziness, light-headedness

Nervousness, depression, and irritability

Blurred vision

Overwhelming fatigue

Panic attacks

Pounding heart, palpitations, or irregular heartbeat

Severe anxiety

Trembling of the hands, "butterflies in the stomach"

Flushing and/or sweating

Faintness or actual fainting

Feeling of pressure in the head, headache in the forehead

Ringing in the ears

Numbness or tingling in the hands, feet, or face

Cramps in the feet and legs

Insomnia

Abdominal pains, gas

Diarrhea

Blood sugar is measured in milligrams of glucose per deciliter (one-hundredth of a liter, about a third of an ounce) of blood, and expressed as a whole number. Normal fasting blood sugars range from 70 to 125 mg/dl. People with fasting blood sugars in this range will begin to show symptoms of hypoglycemia at 50 to 55. A person with a fasting blood glucose in the diabetic range (over 126) may well show symptoms at a level higher than 55.

Hypoglycemia has a multitude of symptoms. They reflect the fact that the brain is being deprived of its primary fuel, glucose.

If you get hungry a couple of hours after a meal, you are experiencing hypoglycemia. If you find yourself becoming irritable or unreasonably angry as mealtime approaches, you are experiencing hypoglycemia. If nightmares often wake you in the middle of the night, they are probably induced by hypoglycemia. Your blood sugar drops suddenly, adrenaline floods your bloodstream in an attempt to bring your glucose level back up, and you wake in terror. The same thing can happen in the daytime, and you think you're having a panic attack. It's as if you have been confronted with sudden danger, only the adrenaline surge comes in response to a drop in blood sugar.

• *ALAN: When I was a child, I'd get light-headed and reach for something sugary. It didn't occur to me that this was abnormal, so I didn't mention it to anyone. In high school I played a lot of sports. I could eat as much sugar as I wanted without any problems. At 148 pounds, I was still thin when I finished high school in 1991. After six months in college, though, I was getting that light-headed feeling again. I began ducking out to McDonald's for french fries almost every day. I was also starting to gain weight.*

Two years later I'd gained more than 50 pounds. My weight was breaking 200 for the first time. I'd start to feel foggy and light-headed, so I'd eat. Then I'd feel really bad and have to lie down for an hour or two, with my heart pounding the whole time. Right after that, I would be hungry again, and the cycle would start over.

Gradually, I began to associate my symptoms with eating sweets and starchy foods. I went to the campus clinic to find out what was wrong with me. The doctor ordered blood tests. The results were within the normal range, except that my HDL [the good kind of blood fat] was 34, far too low. I was twenty-one. My fasting blood sugar was 79, on the low side of normal but nothing to be alarmed about, the doctor said. I told the doctor how sick I felt, and the doctor was annoyed. He said, "Well, you're not diabetic yet, so it's not like insulin would help. If you've noticed that foods like potatoes make you feel bad, then don't eat them." I went back to my room to lie down.

I decided to buy a glucometer, a device for measuring my own blood glucose levels, and began keeping records. After a month I went back to campus health and saw a different doctor. She ordered a glucose tolerance test for later in the week. I thought, Finally, something will be done.

After a twelve-hour fast, I went for the test. The technician drew blood to get a fasting glucose level, then gave me a very sweet soda to drink. They drew blood at thirty minutes, one, two, and three hours. At the two-hour mark, lying on the couch in the waiting room, I wasn't feeling very good at all. I could almost feel myself leaving my body. At three hours, I was shaking very badly. I couldn't think and was verbally combative. After they took their last blood sample, they had to talk me into getting into a wheelchair so they could get me out of the lab and into a room where they could try to figure out what was wrong. A doctor came into the room and said that my two-hour glucose was only 52. However, it had come back up to 84, undoubtedly from the adrenaline released when it got so low. They fed me some glucose tablets and made me promise I would go eat at McDonald's right away.

A week later, I made a follow-up visit to see what the doctor would say. She told me I was definitely hypoglycemic, but had no suggestions about what to do. A nurse in the office suggested I keep packets of grape jelly from McDonald's in my pocket and eat them if my blood sugar got uncomfortably low. While I was happy at least to have a solid diagnosis, I was terribly disappointed in the medical system once again for an utter lack of assistance.

It's hard to understand how a doctor who has seen a hypoglycemic person's reaction to the sugary drink given patients at the beginning of the glucose tolerance test can continue to recommend more starches and sugars to combat a sudden drop in blood sugar. This may be acceptable advice for an insulin-dependent diabetic, whose risk if insulin drives blood glucose too low requires immediate rescue. But even in that case most doctors will suggest a glass of milk rather than fruit juice, unless the diabetic person can't tolerate milk. For someone with reactive hypoglycemia, such advice is equivalent to suggesting alcohol as the remedy for symptoms of alcoholism.

Carbohydrates are not alone in inducing a hypoglycemic episode. Caffeine stimulates the release of the adrenal hormones that cause the liver to release glycogen, raising blood sugar for a quick burst of energy. This signals the pancreas to discharge insulin, which lowers the blood sugar and stimulates the adrenals, and so forth. This is not to suggest, if you are a heavy coffee drinker, that you stop it entirely all at once. The only way to decaffeinate is to do it gradually. The alternative, going cold turkey, will probably induce a headache you will never forget.

Certain other things can trigger hypoglycemic attacks, including certain recreational drugs, marijuana and cocaine chief among them. People who are intolerant of dairy products may experience reactive hypoglycemia after drinking a glass of milk, which contains lactose, or milk sugar. Fructose (fruit sugar), abundant in fruit juice, can also cause a hypoglycemic reaction, which is why it is a mistake to drink fruit juice or anything sweetened with corn syrup (especially high-fructose corn syrup) in response to hypoglycemia. Reactive hypoglycemia associated with lactose or fructose intolerance is often accompanied by vomiting.

What is the role of insulin resistance in hypoglycemia? The final answer is not yet known, but since insulin-resistant people have excessive insulin in their bloodstreams, it is reasonable to conjecture that the insulin overreacts, triggering the cascade of events that hypoglycemics experience. That would explain why reactive hypoglycemia, like insulin resistance, is a hereditary condition.

> • LEN: *Hypoglycemia nearly cost my father his job when I was a kid. Each day after lunch he would buy a big bag of chocolates and eat them all afternoon. One day his boss caught him sleeping at his desk, and things changed quite a bit at work.*
>
> *My dad saw several doctors. None of them could understand his symptoms, until one sent him for a glucose tolerance test. Sure enough, he had it bad. When my dad changed his diet, he was a completely different man.*
>
> *At the same time, I was having lots of problems growing up—restlessness, bad grades, getting into fights. I was in trouble all the time. When I was fifteen, my father took me for a glucose tolerance test. The results were like his. I, too, changed my eating ways. I was thankful to know what was making me so miserable. It's nice to know what your body can and cannot take. I only wish this had been discovered in the early 1900s, when my father's mother was put in a mental ward with exactly the same symptoms. My four-year-old son is just like me, my dad, and my grandmother.*

Unfortunately, physicians often perceive hypoglycemia's symptoms as caused by mental illness and offer mood-altering drugs (antianxiety drugs or, increasingly, antidepressants) or psychotherapy instead of suggesting dietary changes that stand a much better chance of alleviating the problem. If your problem is *reactive* hypoglycemia, the kind that gets worse after eating, with a bit of care and determination you can handle it yourself, without medical intervention. As with many other chronic dysfunctions, the precise answer to your hypoglycemia will reflect the fact that you and your body chemistry are absolutely unique. There is no one-size-fits-all answer. But there are basic principles you can apply. Gradually, you will learn the variations that lead to your success. Here are some suggestions to get you on your way.

Keep a food-mood diary for a week to ten days. Put the date at the top of the page, and record everything that goes into your mouth—food, drink, medications, nutritional supplements, and all—along with the time of day. This will work best if you make your notes at the time you eat or drink, rather than trusting your memory. Measure quantities as much as possible. Eventually you will be able to make accurate estimates, but even when you have gained that skill, it's a good idea to spot-check your estimates occasionally. Note also how you feel, physically and emotionally, each time you eat. And when your mood or physical sensations change—for example, when you get an attack of the blues, or feel suddenly anxious or irritable—note that, too, with the time.

If during this record-keeping period you see a pattern that enables you to relate a specific food to a specific physical or mood change, feel free to drop that substance from your diet, noting in your diary the facts and reasons for the change. The sole exception to this is any medication you are taking. If you find that a prescription drug seems to be having a bad effect, check with the physician who prescribed it before discontinuing it. As to food and drink, though, perhaps scientific method would require that you make no changes during this investigative period, but your primary goal here is relief of your symptoms, not science. Just keep an accurate account of what you are doing and what is happening.

By the end of this test period you are almost sure to have identified at least some of the foods that are causing trouble for you. They may be some of your favorite food items, or things you crave and go out of your way to buy. Generally, people may have two distinct reactions to the information that their favorite foods are making them sick. Some lucky ones, faced with the fact that the food they love best in all the world is their enemy, lose their taste for it entirely. It is perfectly natural, however, to receive this news with a sense of despair and the feeling you can't possibly give the food up entirely. If the substance is coffee, for example, the prudent reaction is to start cutting down, perhaps by mixing regular and decaffeinated coffee at the start, increasing the decaf portion in relation to the regular day by day. Caffeine is one of the most addictive substances in common use. Don't try to give it up cold turkey, but do work on giving it up. If the beverage that is causing the most trouble is beer, wine, or hard liquor, please seek professional help in eliminating it from your diet. Don't be ashamed. Alcohol is a physically addictive substance. It's not an indictment of your character or worth as a human being if you have a problem with alcohol, but it's probably not a problem you can solve without help and support. In fact, if your body is accustomed to large quantities of alcohol on a regular basis, quitting without medical help could have serious consequences.

If you look at your food diary and nothing leaps out at you, then begin by suspecting all the white things you eat—sugar, white flour, white rice, potatoes—and any ingredient in processed foods that ends in -ose: sucrose, dextrose, fructose, lactose, maltose, and glucose. Learn to read lists of ingredients on the labels of processed foods. In the United States, manufacturers are required to list all ingredients in order, by volume, starting with the largest quantity and decreasing as the list goes on. Later in this book you will learn to read the nutrition information labels that report on macronutrients—proteins, carbohydrates, and fats—so that you can fine-tune your way of eating. But for now your best bet is to watch out for the foods most likely to cause your hypoglycemic reaction.

Don't let yourself get hungry. Some hypoglycemics do best on six *small* meals a day; others eat three meals and have small snacks between meals. Snacks should consist of a protein and a fat, not a carbohydrate. Carry with you packets of nuts, seeds, or small cubes of cheese. Among nuts, macadamias, walnuts, and almonds are best. Peanuts and cashews are beans, not nuts, and are a poor choice for hypoglycemics. Keep snack foods of this kind in your desk at work, in the glove compartment of your car, and in your briefcase or handbag. Don't worry about your weight while you're getting your hypoglycemia under control. Chances are you'll lose without trying as you phase out of your life the foods that are causing you trouble, but if you don't, you'll have time later to deal with your weight if you choose.

• *MARY: The first doctor I saw about the symptoms I eventually learned were caused by reactive hypoglycemia told me to drink fruit juice to keep my blood sugar level up. I kept a bottle of apple cider in my office refrigerator and drank juice frequently during the day. It feels stupid to say this now, but I didn't make the connection between the juice and my increasing fatigue and brain fog. Eventually, and it didn't take long, work at a job I loved had become a nightmare. I went to see a doctor who specializes in glandular problems. I needed my husband to come with me because I was having trouble completing a thought and didn't feel safe driving a car.*

The endocrinologist listened to my history and my complaints. He looked at the results of my fasting blood sugar test. It was well within the normal range. He asked me if I was willing to undergo a thirty-six-hour fast and then take a longer glucose tolerance test, one that would last for five hours. I gulped at the thought of a thirty-six-hour fast, but I was desperate, so I agreed.

Believe me, you don't go to work when you're on a thirty-six-hour fast. I started after dinner on a Saturday night and had nothing but water until Monday morning, when I had an appointment at the lab for the glucose tolerance test. During much of the fast I stayed in bed, reading or dozing. The first twelve hours were a snap. I slept most of the time, since the fast started at night. The second twelve hours were a bit difficult, but not nearly as awful as I'd anticipated. By the end of twenty-four hours it was bedtime again, and I slept through the last twelve hours. I felt a bit weak in the morning, but I didn't need help getting to the hospital lab.

The glucose tolerance test was the worst part of the whole experience—not something I'd like to repeat. When I went back to the endocrinologist to hear about the test results, I already knew I had a problem with glucose. That was easy to figure out. During the test I felt worse and worse as the hours passed. During the fourth hour I was shaking with cold. When I got out of the recliner to go ask for a blanket, I fainted.

But the endocrinologist taught me an important lesson by asking me to fast. He explained that he was trying to rule out an insulin-producing tumor. If I'd had such a tumor, he said, I could not have completed the fast. The tumor would have gone right on manufacturing insulin and lowering my blood sugar regardless of what I did or did not eat. He didn't say so right out, but I learned that day that I was better off eating nothing than the wrong things. That knowledge came as a turning point in my life. My task then became figuring out what were the wrong things, and avoiding them.

·5·
DIABETES

THE FOURTH MOST common reason for patients to contact their doctors is diabetes mellitus, or sugar diabetes, a condition in which too much glucose is found in the bloodstream and urine. The surplus of sugar leads to problems with arteries and blood circulation. Diabetic patients are at risk of blindness, neurological problems, heart disease, stroke, and the loss of limbs due to poor circulation. A diabetic's kidneys work overtime to expel the excess sugar, making kidney disease a major risk.

Diabetes is a group of disorders that can be divided into three subtypes. Type 1, or insulin-dependent, diabetes is also known as juvenile onset diabetes, although it sometimes develops in early adulthood. Type 1 diabetes is an autoimmune condition in which the immune system attacks pancreatic cells that produce insulin. Type 1 diabetics typically use injected insulin to control the disease. Type 2, or non-insulin-dependent, diabetes is also known as adult onset diabetes, although a growing number of children are being diagnosed with it. Type 2 is also known as insulin-resistant diabetes. You can be insulin resistant and not diabetic—heredity plays a crucial role here—but Type 2 diabetics are always insulin resistant. The third type is secondary diabetes; that is, diabetes linked to another condition or disorder such as a disease of the pancreas or endocrine system. This book does not deal with secondary diabetes.

GESTATIONAL DIABETES

Gestational diabetes is the term for elevated glucose levels that occur during pregnancy in a woman who was not previously diabetic. It happens in 1 to 2 percent of all pregnancies, usually beginning in the second or third trimester, when pregnancy-associated hormones that are antagonistic to insulin reach their peak levels.[1] The likelihood of developing gestational diabetes increases with age and with each successive pregnancy. The condition usually disappears after delivery. Gestational diabetes has more serious implications for the fetus than for the mother, and physicians take the condition very seriously, although the pregnant woman may show no symptoms other than a slightly elevated blood sugar reading.

Gestational diabetes is a problem of insulin resistance, not a failure of the pancreas to produce insulin. The placenta, the membrane that supplies the fetus with nutrients and water from the mother's body, produces hormones essential to support the pregnancy. It is a paradox that some of these hormones—estrogen and cortisol, among others—interfere with the activity of insulin. Usually the pregnant woman's pancreas is able to produce enough extra insulin to overcome the resistance the placental hormones cause. But in a small percentage of women, there aren't enough beta cells in the pancreas to do the job. After childbirth the placental hormones disappear, and the woman's blood sugar usually returns to normal.

Any woman can develop gestational diabetes, but some factors make it more likely. Obesity is one, as are a family history of diabetes or insulin resistance; a previous pregnancy that resulted in a stillbirth, a child with a birth defect, or a very large newborn; and having too much amniotic fluid. Age is also a factor; as women grow older, the risk increases.

The diagnosis of gestational diabetes is a cause for concern, but not for fear. One thing not to worry about is the possibility

1. J. H. Stein, ed., *Internal Medicine* (Mosby CD Online, 1998).

of birth defects. Almost all birth defects originate during the first trimester of pregnancy—that is, before the thirteenth week. Women who have gestational diabetes usually have normal blood sugar levels during the crucial first trimester; insulin resistance caused by placental hormones rarely occurs before the twenty-fourth week. Nevertheless, careful control of blood glucose levels is essential from the moment the diagnosis of gestational diabetes is confirmed.

The main problem a woman with the diagnosis faces is the possibility that her baby will grow too large in the uterus for a normal vaginal delivery. The developing fetus obtains all of its nutrients directly from the mother's blood. If that blood has too much glucose, the fetus will produce too much insulin in an effort to convert the glucose to energy, and the excess glucose will be converted to fat. If the fetus is too large to pass through the birth canal, a cesarean section is required—not a disaster, but the recovery period is longer than that for a normal birth.

Another risk is that the infant will become hypoglycemic immediately after birth. This happens if the mother's blood sugar level has been high during the third trimester, causing the infant to have high levels of insulin in its bloodstream in response. Since once it is born, the baby no longer receives its mother's high-glucose blood, there is a danger that the newborn's glucose level will drop too low, bringing with it the risk of brain damage. A newborn baby's blood glucose levels are closely monitored from birth. At the first indication of hypoglycemia, intravenous glucose is administered, and the blood sugar level continues under surveillance until the doctor is satisfied that it will remain normal. Hypoglycemic newborns are also vulnerable to certain chemical imbalances, among them deficiencies in calcium and magnesium in the blood.

All of these problems can be prevented and managed. Prevention requires that the mother exercise tight control over her blood sugar levels throughout the rest of her pregnancy, once gestational diabetes is diagnosed. Standard procedure calls for checking blood sugar levels several times a day—commonly before breakfast and two hours after each meal—by a relatively simple procedure that is done at home. If the expectant mother's blood sugar levels remain within normal limits (between 60 and 120 mg/dl), there is less likelihood that the fetus will grow too large, or that the newborn will develop hypoglycemia or chemical imbalances.

If blood sugar tests reveal levels above 120 two hours after eating, the doctor may want to start the woman on insulin by injection, to protect the fetus from being exposed to excessive sugar in the mother's blood. Insulin is given by injection because it is a protein and would be digested like any other protein if taken by mouth.

There is nothing about gestational diabetes that predicts a labor that is anything other than normal, as long as the fetus has not grown too large for vaginal delivery. Control of maternal blood sugar levels must continue during labor. A woman who did not need insulin during pregnancy will not need it during labor or delivery, but a woman who took insulin during pregnancy may be given an insulin injection early in her labor. Sometimes, but not often, intravenous insulin is required throughout labor.

Usually the mother's blood sugar returns to normal as soon as the placenta is delivered. Probably all that will remain to remind the mother that she had gestational diabetes is one more finger stick the morning following delivery, to determine that her blood sugar has indeed returned to normal.

Exercise is a potent tool in keeping gestational diabetes under control. A woman who exercised before becoming pregnant can continue her exercise practices, possibly with a slight decrease in intensity, as explained below. A woman who has been sedentary before pregnancy should begin an exercise program in consultation with her health care practitioner. Among its other benefits, exercise increases the efficiency of insulin—that is, it combats insulin resistance. A good exercise program may prevent gestational diabetes in a woman who would otherwise be prone to developing it.

The only precaution is this: exercise that is too vigorous may direct blood flow away from the uterus and fetus and so should be avoided. According to a report by the American College of Obstetricians and Gynecologists, the target heart rates for pregnant women should be between 25 and 30 percent lower than for nonpregnant women, and in any case should not exceed 140 beats per minute, about 23 beats in 10 seconds.[2]

What about after childbirth? The healthy woman can expect to return to her normal state of health. With the placenta gone, the hormones that caused insulin resistance during pregnancy are also gone, or at least reduced to levels that will not cause insulin resistance. But there is a greater likelihood of gestational diabetes during any subsequent pregnancy. According to Dr. J. H. Stein, one-third to one-half of women with gestational diabetes will develop Type 2 diabetes within five to ten years after childbirth.[3]

Some physicians believe that gestational diabetes develops in women who have too few pancreatic beta cells, the cells that produce insulin. They are therefore unable to generate the additional insulin demanded of them in response to the insulin-resistance-producing placental hormones. A team of researchers headed by Dr. R. K. Peters found that women with gestational diabetes had a 31 percent chance of developing Type 2 diabetes after a subsequent pregnancy, compared with 12 percent for women who have not had gestational diabetes.[4] This suggests that insulin resistance damages beta cells, making diabetes more likely to occur later in life.

2. American College of Obstetricians and Gynecologists, *Home Exercise Program: Exercise During Pregnancy and the Postnatal Period,* May 1985.
3. Stein, *Internal Medicine.*
4. R. K. Peters et al., "Long-Term Diabetogenic Effect of Single Pregnancy in Women with Previous Gestational Diabetes Mellitus," *Lancet* 347 (1996): 227–30.

TYPE 2 DIABETES

Also known as adult onset or insulin-resistant diabetes, Type 2 diabetes is by far the most common form of the disease. Some 85 to 90 percent of diabetics have this form. Type 2 diabetics are insulin resistant. Their cells do not respond to insulin. As far as glucose is concerned, the cell doors are locked, so glucose remains in the bloodstream. The pancreas responds by trying harder, secreting even more insulin. The result is that Type 2 diabetics have both too much sugar and too much insulin in their blood.

Type 2 diabetes usually appears after age forty and is most commonly associated with obesity. This is not to say that obesity is invariably the cause of Type 2 diabetes. There's a chicken-egg question here, and the answer is probably that obesity feeds insulin resistance as much as insulin resistance feeds obesity.

> • *BARBARA: My husband Bert is one of those people who never gets sick and never misses work. My first clue something was wrong was when he missed two days of work. The next week, he missed three; the week after, two more. We soon realized that he still had the flu we'd had together a month ago. He was very thirsty and began drinking huge quantities of soft drinks, Gatorade, and water. He had no appetite and just forced himself to eat. When I took him to the doctor, he was extremely weak. He had a high fever and abdominal pain. The weight was just dropping off him, no matter how much or what he ate. He switched from diet drinks to regular ones, but still couldn't keep his weight up. When the doctor did a blood test, his blood sugar was close to 800. The doctor said Type 2.*

Insulin-resistant people can be Type 2 diabetics for years before they are diagnosed. Bert's case was unusual. The classic symptoms of diabetes—unquenchable thirst, excessively frequent urination, unexplained weight loss, and overwhelming fatigue—are often mild or even absent in Type 2 diabetics. The disease may not be detected until one of the typical complications of diabetes appears. Screening for diabetes is one of the best reasons imaginable to have a periodic physical checkup. Hyperglycemia—excess sugar in the blood—is the decisive finding.

The table shows the typical progression from normal status to Type 2 diabetes. Not everyone goes as far as diabetes, though. Many individuals stop at one of the earlier stages. Heredity, body mass index, and the level of physical activity are the deciding factors.

PROGRESSION FROM NORMAL STATUS TO TYPE 2 DIABETES.

Status	Blood glucose	Blood insulin
Normal	Normal	Normal
Stage 1	Normal	Elevated (hyperinsulinemia)
Stage 2	Elevated (impaired glucose tolerance)	Elevated (hyperinsulinemia)
Stage 3	High (Type 2 diabetes)	Elevated (hyperinsulinemia)

Epidemiologists, the people who keep track of the prevalence of various diseases, estimate that between 3 and 5 percent of the U.S. population has Type 2 diabetes. The prevalence climbs to 10 to 15 percent among people past fifty years of age. It is more common and occurs at an earlier age among Native Americans, people of Mexican descent, and African Americans.

Both obesity and Type 2 diabetes are found in increasing numbers among people from India, Polynesia, and Micronesia when they adopt Western lifestyles. The same is true of people of Japanese descent who have emigrated to the United States. Since insulin resistance is associated with both obesity and Type 2 diabetes, it makes sense to consider insulin resistance as the common denominator in increasing occurrence of both conditions among these ethnic groups, whose lifestyles changed so radically when they moved into Western society. Even the American Dietetic Association—advocate of a high-carbohydrate diet for everyone, including those afflicted with diabetes—acknowledges that a "Westernized" lifestyle is associated with an increased frequency of Type 2 diabetes. That organization, however, is unable to reach consensus on the reason for the dramatic upswing in cases of insulin resistant diabetes in children. Until recently, the association says in a 1999 consensus report on diabetes in children, 98 percent of diabetic children had the autoimmune Type 1 form of the disease, and only 2 percent had the insulin-resistant form. Recent reports, however, indicate that the percentage of Type 2 diagnoses in children under age eighteen has risen to 45 percent. The American Diabetes Association in its 1999 consensus statement ascribed the increase to a more sedentary lifestyle (which is certainly part of the problem) and increased intake of fat. The association completely ignored overconsumption of carbohydrates as a possibility.[5]

This is not to discount the role of heredity in determining who will become diabetic and who will not. Some people can be both insulin resistant and obese their entire lives yet never develop diabetes. The likelihood that a person will become diabetic is greatly increased if one or both parents are diabetic.

There is a relationship between gestational diabetes and increased risk of diabetes in the offspring in adulthood.[6] This should come as no surprise, since excess fat is associated with insulin resistance. The irony is that people on the bottom third of the scale for birth weight—so-called low-birth-weight babies—

5. American Diabetes Association, "Consensus Statement: Type 2 Diabetes in Children and Adolescents," 1999.
6. Gerald M. Reaven and Ami Laws, eds., *Insulin Resistance: The Metabolic Syndrome X* (Totowa, N.J.: Humana Press, 1999), p. 36.

also have an increased risk of diabetes in adulthood. A study at the London School of Hygiene and Tropical Medicine found that sixty-year-old men who at birth were in the bottom fifth on a scale that calculated the percentage of body fat were three times as likely to have diabetes as those who were more well padded.[7]

Today's adolescents may be particularly vulnerable to becoming insulin resistant and developing Type 2 diabetes. The American Diabetes Association theorizes that adolescent insulin resistance is a result of temporary increases in growth hormone, which is secreted by the pituitary gland. When growth hormone is given to adolescents who don't need it, the normal action of insulin deteriorates. Thus, the organization says, "increased growth hormone secretion is most likely responsible for the insulin resistance during puberty, and both growth hormone secretion and insulin resistance decline with completion of puberty." An overweight adolescent with a family history of diabetes is particularly vulnerable to glucose intolerance and diabetes.

Before manufactured insulin was introduced in 1921 as a means of controlling diabetes, diabetics were told to limit their carbohydrates to 4 percent of their total caloric intake, or 20 grams of carbohydrates (80 calories) in a 2,000-calorie diet. This approach was successful for most people with diabetes, reducing the incidence of side effects such as high blood pressure and blindness.[8]

The introduction of insulin led physicians to ease up on the carbohydrate restriction, first to about 20 percent of total calories (100 carbohydrate grams in a 2,000-calorie diet.) The recommended carbohydrate intake has been increasing ever since. B. Frank Scholl, M.D., must have felt that he was shouting into the wind when he wrote in a 1939 article addressed to diabetics,

---

7. Sharon Begley, "Shaped by Life in the Womb," *Newsweek*, 27 September 1999.
8. Maria Kalergis, Danièle Pacaud, and Jean-François Yale, "Attempts to Control the Glycemic Response to Carbohydrate in Diabetes Mellitus: Overview and Practical Implications." Canadian Journal of Diabetes Care 22, no.1 (1998): 20–29.

"General Rules: avoid all sugars and reduce starches to a mini-mum. Increase the amount of meats and especially oils and fats."[9] In the 1970s 40 percent of calories from carbohydrates (200 grams) was the accepted standard. Since the 1980s it has been about 60 percent, the same as the American Dietetic Associa-tion/U.S. Department of Agriculture's food pyramid, which also prescribes 20 percent each for proteins and fats. With its one-size-fits-all recommendations, the pyramid makes no distinction be-tween diet for diabetic and nondiabetic individuals. Nor does it take insulin resistance or glucose intolerance into account.

Conventional wisdom seems to be undergoing another shift, although not yet in significant numbers in the United States. A report in the *Canadian Journal of Diabetes* says the relative pro-portions of macronutrients is undergoing new scrutiny. In fact, a type of fat known as monounsaturated fat is being considered as a valid alternative to carbohydrate as a source of energy. The ar-ticle says that studies that have explored replacing some of the recommended carbohydrate intake with monounsaturated fat appear to have seen good results.[10]

Another departure from the conventional high-carbohydrate diet recommended for diabetics is the practice of carbohydrate counting. At last we are seeing some clinicians recognizing the primary role of carbohydrates in determining blood sugar re-sponse after meals—a concept that seemed to disappear after the introduction of injectable insulin. Carbohydrate counting was one of four meal-planning approaches used in the American Di-abetes Association's 1998 Diabetes Control and Complications Trial, and was found to be effective in helping patients meet their glucose control goals. It also won praise for allowing flexibility in food choices.[11]

9. B. Frank Scholl, M.D., *Library of Health* (Philadelphia: Historical Publish-ing Co., 1939), p. 1065.
10. Kalergis, "Attempts to Control."
11. Sandra J. Gillespie, Karmeen D. Kulkarni, and Anne E. Daly, "Using Carbo-hydrate Counting in Diabetes Clinical Practice," *Journal of the American Dietetic Association* 98 (August 1998): 8.

·6·
POLYCYSTIC OVARIAN SYNDROME

P ERHAPS NO CONDITION associated with insulin resistance causes as much heartache as polycystic ovarian syndrome (PCOS, also known as Stein-Leventhal syndrome and chronic anovulatory hyperandrogenism), a disorder that affects approximately 6 percent of women who have not reached menopause. As if it weren't bad enough that this disease causes infertility, it is also usually accompanied by physical characteristics that can damage self-esteem.

Women with PCOS are almost invariably insulin resistant and are often obese. If they menstruate at all, their periods are apt to be irregular. Glucose intolerance and high serum triglycerides are also common features of this condition. Women with PCOS have an unusually high risk of diabetes and heart disease. Endometrial cancer (cancer of the lining of the uterus) is a risk for women who do not menstruate. Like other conditions associated with insulin resistance, women with polycystic ovaries tend to have mothers and sisters with the condition as well.

• *ELAINE: I put on about fifty pounds in a few months after I graduated from high school. My menstrual periods stopped, and I began growing hair in inappropriate places. The growth of facial hair was bloody embarrassing. It took me four years to get up the courage to see a gynecologist. When I did, in 1988, he said my problem was that I was fat. He offered to prescribe a drug that suppresses male hormones to stop the hair growth. I told him, "A razor is cheaper, and it doesn't have side effects."*

Ten years later I started having vaginal spotting almost every day. When the spotting turned to heavy bleeding, I was frightened. It was then that I learned from my primary physician that the gynecologist I'd seen in 1988 had discovered cysts on my ovaries but hadn't told me about them. My primary doctor did another ultrasound and some blood tests. He, too, saw cystic ovaries, and the blood work was what you'd find with polycystic ovarian syndrome.

I went to a different gynecologist and asked him for birth control pills to regulate my periods. The doctor refused because I smoke cigarettes, and the doctor said the combination of hormones and nicotine can be harmful. He took specimens for a biopsy. The verdict was endometrial cancer. I had my uterus and ovaries surgically removed.

I didn't mind skipping menstrual periods, but now that I understand the connection between lack of menstruation and the risk of endometrial cancer, I feel differently about that.

After I was diagnosed with PCOS and found out that obesity is linked to it through hyperinsulinemia, my mother told me that she could never understand why I was so much heavier than my sisters when I ate less than they did. Now we both know.

There is little agreement in the medical community as to whether insulin resistance causes PCOS, although many doctors are quite willing to blame obesity. In at least one study, nonobese women with PCOS were more likely to have features of the insulin-resistance syndrome (including a waist-to-hip ratio of 0.8 or more, higher fasting insulin and blood glucose levels, and elevated triglycerides) than healthy women of equal body mass index and age.[1]

1. Ingvar Ek, et al., "Impaired Adipocyte Lipolysis in Nonobese Women with the Polycystic Ovary Syndrome: A Possible Link to Insulin Resistance?," *Journal of Clinical Endocrinology and Metabolism* 82 (1997): 1147–53.

The argument in favor of insulin resistance as the cause of PCOS is this: In women, high blood insulin levels increase the adrenal gland's secretion of the androgen hormones (testosterone, androsterone, and DHEA). Although androgens are thought of as male hormones, they are present in women, too, just as the estrogenic hormones (estradiol, estriol, and estrone) are present in men. Women with PCOS have excess male hormones circulating in their blood. This causes the growth of hair on the face and chest, as well as male-pattern baldness, the thinning of hair on the top of the head. Receptors for insulin and insulin-like growth factor 1 (IGF-1) are found in the ovaries. When these receptors are overstimulated, they become extra-sensitive to sex hormones. Excessive secretion of male hormones also interferes with ovulation, which is the cause of infertility in PCOS.

There is a class of drugs known as oral antihyperglycemic agents. Metformin (brand name Glucophage) is one such drug. Reducing insulin resistance with such medications reduces androgen levels in obese women with PCOS, often with a resulting relief of menstrual problems, according to Dr. Richard S. Legro in the *American Journal of Obstetrics and Gynecology*.[2] This is another reason to think that insulin resistance is an important part of the cause of PCOS.

High levels of androgens in women cause fat to be deposited in the male pattern, in the front of the body and especially above the waist (the apple shape), rather than in the hip and pelvic area (the pear shape), as is more normal in women. This link between the distribution of fat and the symptoms associated with insulin resistance suggests that there is something about the way fat cells store triglycerides that affects the development of disorders related to insulin resistance, including PCOS. Fat cells use an enzyme called lipase to store triglycerides for future use when glucose stores are low. (When you see a medical term ending

2. Richard S. Legro, M.D., "Polycystic Ovary Syndrome: Current and Future Treatment Paradigms," *American Journal of Obstetrics and Gynecology* 179 (1998): S101–108.

with *-ase*, you know you're reading about an enzyme. Enzymes are proteins that can produce chemical changes in other substances without being changed themselves.) Lipolysis is the process by which fats are released. The adrenal stress hormones stimulate lipolysis; insulin holds it back, keeping the fat in the cells rather than letting it escape and be burned for energy. If you are insulin resistant, not only do you tend to store more fat in the first place, but you also have to deal with the consequences of insulin preventing you from burning it when you need it. Dr. Legro found that women with PCOS showed as much as a 40 percent lower response to the stress hormones causing the breakdown of fats than did healthy women, whether or not the PCOS women were obese.[3]

Although studies have not established it beyond doubt, considerable evidence supports the idea that PCOS in a young woman signals a significant risk of cardiovascular disease later in life, providing another link between insulin resistance and PCOS. Chest pain in young women with PCOS is more likely to be related to coronary artery disease than it would be in the average young woman. According to Dr. Ann E. Taylor, any symptom that might be related to cardiovascular disease should be taken more seriously in women with PCOS than in the general population.[4]

About 40 percent of women with PCOS do not ovulate at all. Dr. David Guzick found that when these women are able to ovulate, about 80 percent of them become pregnant within the first nine regular menstrual cycles.[5]

Because ovaries produce progesterone only after ovulation, women with PCOS are often exposed solely to estrogen, without

---

3. Legro, "Polycystic Ovary Syndrome."
4. Ann E. Taylor, M.D., "Understanding the Underlying Metabolic Abnormalities of Polycystic Ovary Syndrome and Their Implications," *American Journal of Obstetrics and Gynecology* 179 (1998): S94–100.
5. David Guzick, M.D., "Polycystic Ovary Syndrome: Symptomatology, Pathophysiology, and Epidemiology," *American Journal of Obstetrics and Gynecology* 179 (1998): S89–93.

progesterone to balance it. This poses the danger of en-
dometriosis (an overgrowth into the abdomen of the lining of
the womb) and endometrial cancer. Women who do not ovulate
should be monitored carefully by means of Pap smears, ultrasound of the uterus, or both.

Some 74 percent of women with PCOS are diagnosed when
they see their doctors for help with infertility. The doctor may
decide to treat the symptom (infertility) rather than the cause
(PCOS) by using drugs to stimulate ovulation. The excess of
male hormones associated with PCOS makes these women especially susceptible to overstimulation of the ovaries, resulting in
multiple births.

·7·

CANDIDIASIS

ANDIDA IS the genus name for a yeast that normally inhabits the digestive and urinary-genital tracts of human beings. There are some 150 species of *Candida;* the most common is *C. albicans.* In this discussion I'll use the words *candida* and *yeast* interchangeably.

One of the common myths about candidiasis is that only women get it, and then only as vaginal yeast. This misconception is unfortunate, even dangerous, because yeast overgrowth can cause a host of ailments and can even be life threatening. Its effects are confined neither to vaginas nor to women.

Under normal circumstances we live in a symbiotic relationship with our yeasts. That is, they cannot live without us, and we cannot live without them. We share our food with them. In return, they guard us from any harmful bacteria that find their way into our intestines. Millions of them inhabit our intestines when we are healthy, their numbers kept in check by the "friendly" bacteria that also live inside us.

However, when things go awry, we can become victims of our yeast population. The condition that results is known as candidiasis or systemic yeast overgrowth. Several things can happen that allow our yeasts to grow out of control. The one that concerns us most here is insulin resistance, but there are other factors of which you should be aware.

Anything that compromises your immune system, including excessive stress and steroid hormones, can make your internal environment friendly to the proliferation of yeast. Chronic candidiasis is common among diabetics, people with HIV disease/AIDS, and those who have undergone chemotherapy to treat cancer. Commonly used medical interventions can throw your system out of balance and provide a fertile field in which candida can overgrow. Steroids weaken the immune system; that's why they are used to combat autoimmune diseases. Antibiotics, taken to kill harmful bacterial invaders, also kill off the friendly bacteria that keep candida in check. Estrogen replacement therapy interferes with the normal bacterial balance in the gut as well. While steroids, antibiotics, and estrogen may at times be necessary to combat serious ailments, you should be aware of their potential harm to your yeast balance and take steps to maintain that balance as best you can.

Probiotics such as acidophilus and bifidus, the friendly bacteria that keep yeast in check, can be found in health food stores. There, too, you will find other substances such as caprylic acid and oil of garlic, which are toxic to yeast and can help you overcome candidiasis. Books and Internet resources dedicated to dealing with yeast overgrowth are listed in the bibliography and appendix 3.

People with diabetes are another group especially vulnerable to yeast overgrowth. High levels of glucose in the blood provide candida with the nourishment it needs to grow out of control. Your blood glucose doesn't have to be at the diabetic level to encourage yeast overgrowth; you need only be insulin resistant and eat a diet high in carbohydrates.

When conditions favor the rapid multiplication of yeasts, candida changes from a single-cell fungus to a form that branches and spreads, and begins to invade the entire body. Much as some forms of grass grow by putting out rhizomes—branches that reach out and away from the mother plant—yeast can put out long, rootlike structures that escape from the intestines by punching microscopic holes in the intestinal walls, allowing yeast, undigested food particles, bacteria, and other toxic wastes to enter the bloodstream. This can give rise to leaky gut syndrome, involved in both malnutrition and various autoimmune diseases (see chapter 9).

Candida that has escaped from the digestive tract can set up in other parts of the body. Among common sites are the bladder, causing chronic bladder infections (cystitis); and the nasal sinuses, causing chronic sinusitis. Many allergies have their origin in yeast overgrowth. Candidiasis is implicated in tinnitus, a condition in which there is a constant buzzing or ringing in the ears. It is also involved in some cases of hearing loss.

> • *MIRYAM: In 1993 I began having a series of episodes in which my hearing suddenly diminished, then returned gradually over a period of days. Each time I was left with slightly less ability to hear than I previously had. My otologist [a specialist in diseases of the ear and hearing] ruled out everything he could think of: autoimmune inner ear disease and tumor on the acoustic nerve. In 1996 I got my hearing aids. The doctor said they would help me for about five years, but after that I'd be beyond the help of hearing aids.*
>
> *I could not accept the idea of losing the ability to hear music and the spoken word. I started doing my own research in the medical literature. Luckily I had learned the medical term for my kind of hearing loss: fluctuating sensorineural hearing loss. Searching the archives of the National Library of Medicine, I found hundreds of references. All but one were about the two conditions the doctor had ruled out. The exception referred to an article on the use of Nystatin, an antifungal drug, to treat hearing loss. The paper had not been published because it reported on a number of cases, not a clinical study. Such articles are looked down upon in the medical community as being unscientific. No journal was willing to publish the paper, but an editorial in one journal gave a brief overview of the treatment and encouraged*

physicians to investigate it.[1] I managed to locate the doctor who had written it and get the report. It told of some twenty people whose hearing loss had been halted when they took Nystatin oral powder dissolved in water for two months, along with what the paper referred to as "dietary control," without going into detail. The paper did not go so far as to say that the hearing loss was caused by fungal growth in the ears, but the inference was inescapable.

I tried the Nystatin treatment for two months and stopped. Two months later I had another episode of lost hearing. I started Nystatin again, this time with a rigorous yeast elimination diet, guessing that was what the author of the paper meant by dietary control. For a few days I felt as though I had a mild case of the flu. I was achy, slightly nauseated, and fatigued—sick enough to contemplate quitting the regimen—but the thought of going totally deaf kept me going. I later learned that the way I felt was perfectly normal, and was caused by the dying yeasts circulating in my bloodstream on the way to being eliminated. Soon the sick feeling left me. I noticed that I was losing weight at a gratifyingly rapid rate (which was fine, as I had plenty to spare) and that my energy level was increasing remarkably. I stayed on the Nystatin regimen for six months, a duration I chose somewhat arbitrarily, having no one to guide me but a doctor sufficiently impressed with my results that she was willing to prescribe Nystatin for as long as I wanted it. I followed the yeast elimination diet for three months, then started looking for something to replace it because it was becoming oppressively restrictive. That's when I discovered low-carbohydrate eating. I've been low-carbing since then.

By my hearing doctor's estimate I should be almost totally deaf by now. My hearing hasn't deteriorated at all since I started the yeast elimination regimen in 1997. And I no longer have any symptoms of yeast overgrowth.

1. J. G. Neely and R. A. Nelson, "Orally Ingested Nystatin Powder in Water for the Stabilization of Hearing in Patients with Fluctuating Hearing Loss," *Otolaryngology—Head and Neck Surgery* 111, no. 1 (July 1994): 1.

·8·

DIGESTIVE DISTURBANCES

EVEN PEOPLE who have trouble accepting the relationship between what they eat and the condition of their arteries and bones can hardly deny the effect of dietary choices on the health of their digestive tract. "It must have been something I ate" is a common cliché, proving the point. "Onions [or cucumbers, or garlic, or some other common food] don't agree with me," we say, stifling a belch. But we never blame the real culprit, an excess of carbohydrates. People who overindulge in sweets and starchy carbohydrates are the ones most vulnerable to insulin resistance. Thus, chronic digestive disturbance may serve as an early warning sign for insulin resistance. The dietary changes that control insulin resistance are most likely to eliminate digestive problems.

HEARTBURN AND GERD

People swallow antacids, pills designed to coat the stomach lining and reduce the caustic affect of gastric juices, often without wondering why they must do so. Advertisements by the makers of antacids have convinced several generations that heartburn is one of those everyday nuisances for which there is but one cure: their product.

• *JIM: I was a strict vegetarian for eight years in an attempt to improve my health. My wife and I had been vegans, no animal products at all, for the last two years. I didn't want anything to do with eating meat. I thought if I was as sick as I was eating vegetarian, I would be really messed up eating meat. As a vegetarian I always had indigestion and a lot of gas. I had been told that meat sat in your bowels for months and rotted, which is why it was so bad for you.*

Chronic heartburn, occurring more than three times a week, is called gastroesophageal reflux disease (GERD). Left untreated, GERD can lead to ulceration, asthma, and narrowing of the food passageway. GERD that continues for several years can lead to Barrett's esophagus, a condition in which cells from the stomach grow into the esophagus. This may actually be a protective device on the part of the body to protect the esophagus from acid that the stomach cells can tolerate but the cells lining the esophagus cannot. People whose long-standing GERD symptoms diminish without explanation should suspect Barrett's esophagus. The condition cannot be reversed, although dietary changes can prevent it from getting worse. People with Barrett's esophagus have a high risk of esophageal cancer.

Heartburn has a simple cause that can often be remedied by a change in diet. When you sit down to eat, even before the first forkful of food reaches your mouth, your digestive system has started working. Anticipating proteins, your stomach starts secreting hydrochloric acid, a substance so caustic it can dissolve glass. Its purpose is to activate the enzymes that break down proteins into nutrients your body can use. If what your stomach gets is a mass of carbohydrates instead, your dinner goes through the stomach into the small intestine so quickly that the acid has little to do, and since your intestine is already full of food, the hydrochloric acid backs up into the esophagus, where it doesn't belong. The pain that results can mimic a heart attack. But it's not your heart that's burning; it's the sensitive tissues of the esophagus. Heartburn isn't caused by too much stomach acid, as the antacid vendors would have us believe. It's caused by acid in the wrong place. Only a few people who have a condition called Zollinger-Ellis syndrome (ZE) actually secrete too much hydrochloric acid. The opposite problem is far more common, particularly in older people.

In addition to deemphasizing carbohydrates in the diet, you can make certain changes in your behavior that will help you to avoid heartburn. Alcohol and caffeine make it worse. Abdominal fat and tight clothing can put pressure on the stomach, forcing undigested food and stomach acid backward into the esophagus. You can make gravity work for you by not lying down for two or three hours after eating, and by using cinder blocks to elevate the head of your bed by six to eight inches. Above all, stop eating before you feel full, eating smaller meals more often, if necessary.

CELIAC DISEASE (NONTROPICAL SPRUE) AND IRRITABLE BOWEL

Without recognizing it, many people are sensitive to gluten, the protein portion of cereal grains such as wheat, oats, rye, and barley. The resulting symptoms are known as gluten-induced enteropathy, celiac disease, or nontropical sprue. (Tropical sprue is something else entirely, thought to be caused by a bacterial infection.) It is a common misconception that celiac sprue is confined to children. It can develop at any time, and 25 percent of those who develop it are past seventy. Sometimes in these people the first symptom is iron-deficiency anemia, caused by associated internal bleeding.

In people with this sensitivity, eating foods containing gluten causes the lining of the small intestine to swell, preventing nutrients from being properly absorbed. One result is a deficiency in B vitamins, which can cause nerve pain, joint aches and pains, anemia, swelling, and skin disorders. Other symptoms of nontropical sprue include abdominal pain and distension, unexplained weight loss, and diarrhea that may at times be bloody.

Celiac sprue is often mistaken for irritable bowel syndrome, a term for any irritation of the bowel for which a cause cannot be found. Like sprue, symptoms of irritable bowel include bloating, abdominal gas, and loose, often urgent bowel movements. Unlike sprue, irritable bowel syndrome sometimes alternates between diarrhea and constipation. If you are suffering from chronic diarrhea that has no explanation, it is best to rule out sprue before assuming it's irritable bowel syndrome. Do this by going on a gluten-free diet for a month to six weeks. If symptoms disappear, that's not proof that it's sprue, because irritable bowel is likely to improve on a low-carbohydrate diet, too. You prove the existence of sprue by adding gluten in small quantities back into your diet. If the symptoms return, you know what is causing them. A small amount of gluten-containing carbohydrate won't be likely to trigger irritable bowel symptoms, but large amounts of carbohydrate when you're testing for sprue will confuse the issue.

Irritable bowel syndrome probably results from a variety of stimuli, but the most common is carbohydrate overload. Carbohydrates move rapidly from the stomach to the small intestine, where they are supposed to be digested into glucose. If you eat more carbohydrates than your system can handle, however, some will escape undigested into the large intestine, where bacteria will break them down into gas, causing pain and distension. In order to dilute the large quantity of sugar in the large intestine, water is pulled out of the bloodstream, causing loose stools.

People who have sprue must avoid foods made with the grains that contain gluten, but often that isn't enough. Many prepared foods contain gluten as a thickener, but food manufacturers are not required to list gluten as a separate ingredient, the way they must list flour and sugar. For people with sprue, there is really no alternative to avoiding all carbohydrates except those found in vegetables and, with moderation, fruits.

INFLAMMATORY BOWEL DISEASES

Ulcerative colitis and Crohn's disease are conditions in which parts of the digestive tract become inflamed, causing abdominal pain, cramping, and diarrhea. They are hard to tell apart, except that ulcerative colitis is confined to the large intestine and rectum; Crohn's disease can show up anywhere from the mouth to the rectum. Most commonly it is found in the small and/or large intestines. Diarrhea is usually bloody in ulcerative colitis. Bleeding is less common with Crohn's disease. Characteristically, the person who has either of these diseases feels an urgent need to get to the toilet shortly after eating, a fact that interferes greatly with normal life and activities.

Chronic diarrhea causes partially digested food to pass through the colon faster than it should. Since the small intestine is where much of the absorption of nutrients from food takes place, too-rapid transit robs the body of needed vitamins and minerals, and deficiencies may result. Also, the large intestine normally absorbs much of the water in the slurry of digested food and wastes. Diarrhea, therefore, is quite likely to cause dehydration. Both develop most commonly in the late teens and twenties, but there is a second peak of occurrences at around age seventy.

The medical literature doesn't have much to say about the cause of inflammatory bowel disease. In extreme cases, doctors prescribe steroids to give relief from symptoms caused by inflammation. Many prescribe antibiotics on the theory that infection is present. This is probably true, but steroids and antibiotics may be exactly the wrong substances to bring about a cure. Sufferers who attack the problem as one of yeast overgrowth and the proliferation of harmful intestinal bacteria are quite often successful in curing themselves.

Inflammatory bowel disease may actually begin with a course of antibiotics or steroids prescribed for good reason—bacterial infection or inflammation that can't be dealt with effectively in any other way. But the most commonly prescribed antibiotics kill virtually every kind of bacteria they come across, including the friendly ones that keep harmful bacteria and intestinal yeast under control. The main purpose of steroids is to weaken the immune system, suspected in inflammatory conditions of conducting an autoimmune attack. When the immune system is weakened, there is less resistance to the takeover by harmful bacteria. So a course of steroids may trigger the need for a course of antibiotics and vice versa, in a vicious cycle that is difficult to bring to an end.

Probably even more common as a cause of inflammatory bowel disease is a dietary emphasis on carbohydrates that gives the small intestine more work than it can handle, leaving bits and pieces of undigested carbohydrates to ferment, damaging the intestinal lining. Yeast and most bacteria require carbohydrates for energy so that they can multiply. When they become dominant, their wastes produce acids and toxins that can further injure the intestinal walls, destroying enzymes required for digestion. Often the walls of the intestine will secrete an overabundance of mucus in an attempt to protect the damaged tissue and help it to heal. When this happens, it is quite common for the stools to be streaked with mucus, a disconcerting phenomenon and a sign that the intestines are in distress.

Another possible explanation of the role of excessive carbohydrate intake in inflammatory bowel disease and other forms of digestive distress has to do with the fact that the pancreas produces a whole army of digestive hormones, not only insulin and glucagon. An increased demand for one of these hormones triggers an increased release of many of the others, so that when a large influx of carbohydrates calls for large amounts of insulin—and in the case of insulin resistance, an extra-large amount—the other hormones, some of them highly acidic, come along for the ride.

Ulcerative colitis that lasts for ten to fifteen years can develop into cancer. To prevent this, surgery is a last-ditch intervention. Gastroenterologist Dr. Wolfgang Lutz says that between 20 and

30 percent of sufferers who don't modify their way of eating require surgery removing the colon and rectum and replacing them with an artificial anus and a bag into which to empty wastes.[1]

When people with inflammatory bowel disease drastically cut their carbohydrate intake, their digestive system distress diminishes or disappears, only to return if they resume their former way of eating. By some accounts, Crohn's disease can be cured on a low-carbohydrate diet followed for a long enough time. Wolfgang Lutz, who followed sixty-seven Crohn's disease patients for three years of low-carbohydrate eating, wrote that 70 percent were symptom free after six months on the diet, and more than 85 percent had no symptoms after eighteen months.[2]

1. Wolfgang Lutz, M.D., *Dismantling a Myth: The Role of Fat and Carbohydrates in Our Diet* (Munich: Selecta-Verlag, 1986), 7.
2. Christian B. Allan and Wolfgang Lutz, *Life without Bread* (Los Angeles: Keats Publishing, 2000), p. 119.

·9·

AUTOIMMUNE DISEASES

Autoimmune diseases are those in which the body attacks a part of itself, rather than being invaded by an infectious outsider. A proposed mechanism for autoimmune disease suggests that the conventional Western diet is at the root of some forms of autoimmunity.

Although you cannot cure yourself of a chronic autoimmune disease by modifying your diet, there is evidence to suggest that you can improve your condition. Indeed, some people consider their autoimmune diseases to be in permanent remission as long as they do what it takes to feel well. The damage autoimmune disease has done is not likely to be reversed, but perhaps your condition will not grow worse, which is no small thing when you're dealing with an autoimmune disease that is causing the destruction of some part of your body.

> • *Kea: I knew something was wrong with me from the time I was fourteen. I spent the summer at camp. When I went to bed at night, my arms and legs would start twitching and keep me from falling asleep. It wasn't happening to anyone else. I also had numbness and cramping in my hands and feet. And I was so easily tired. I couldn't go to the mall with my friends. I couldn't understand how they could stand and walk for so long. When I had to wait for the school bus, I'd take off my coat and use it for a cushion so I could sit. The teachers at the bus line would yell at me.*

My mother took me to doctor after doctor. They ruled out juvenile rheumatoid arthritis and mononucleosis. They said I was perfectly fine, except for those imaginary symptoms.

I got married at nineteen. I had times of terrible fatigue, but no diagnosis. My husband raced harness horses; we had thirty horses in the stable to care for and train. A horse I was riding slipped and fell on me, all 800 pounds of it. It broke my pelvis in seven places. I was in traction for three months. By the time I was twenty-one, with two children, my fatigue was overwhelming. I felt that my legs were encased in cement. I didn't have enough strength to hold a book.

Then, at twenty-three, I lost the sight in my left eye. I went with my mother to an eye doctor who said it was retrobulbar neuritis. He told us that 99 percent of the time, people who have that have multiple sclerosis. Then he left the room. Neither my mother nor I knew what MS was, and we feared it was something that would kill me quickly. When the doctor came back into the examining room, he had made an appointment for me with a neurologist.

The neurologist wanted to do a spinal tap, but I refused because of the damage to my pelvis and the advice of my obstetrician, who delivered my babies by cesarean section, saying a spinal anesthetic wouldn't be safe. The doctor wouldn't give me a diagnosis without a spinal tap. Two years later I went to a major medical center where they did an MRI and other diagnostic tests. I finally knew what was wrong: it was MS. I was twenty-five.

Now I'm forty. I have the relapsing-remitting type of MS. The symptoms come and go. When I was twenty-eight, for a time I was almost completely paralyzed and had to stay in bed. Other times I'm able to exercise the horses and walk in the woods. Mostly I conserve my energy so I can make supper and do normal wife-and-mother things.

Autoimmune diseases are degenerative by nature. That is, tissue is destroyed. Cartilage or bone may be worn away. Among the autoimmune diseases are rheumatoid arthritis, in which inflammation causes deforming changes in the joints; multiple sclerosis, which involves destruction of the myelin sheath, the fatty tissue that surrounds nerves of the central nervous system; systemic lupus erythematosus, an inflammatory disease of connective tissue; and Type 1 diabetes, in which the insulin-producing cells of the pancreas come under attack. Allergy, while not an autoimmune disease, is another type of malfunction of the immune system. Much of the information concerning autoimmunity is pertinent to allergy as well.

Part of your body's wisdom is the ability to recognize what is part of you and what is not. That is the job of your immune system—to differentiate between "self" and "nonself" and get rid of the "nonself" before it harms you. Your body is constantly being invaded by viruses, bacteria, and other foreign substances. Under normal circumstances, your immune system identifies them as "nonself," produces antibodies to them, and eliminates them. If your immune system cannot fight back against invading germs—the influenza virus, for example—because it is weakened or overwhelmed, then you become ill. People who get yearly flu shots are injected with antigens to the strains of influenza virus expected to be most common in the coming year. These antigens stimulate the activity of cells in the lymph system known as B lymphocytes, or B cells, which produce antibodies when the virus invades.

Foreign, "nonself" antigens are not the only ones that attach themselves to the body's cells and attract the attention of the B cells. There are also autoantigens, tags on the cell surface that say, "This cell belongs to this body," and announce what kind of cell it is. Scientists think that as a fetus develops, its immune system cells are exposed to the autoantigens of newly formed cells and learn to recognize them as part of the self.

Sometimes the immune system fails to recognize the autoantigen labels and instead declares war on the cells it perceives as invaders. This is the autoimmune response. If the mistake happens in response to autoantigens on cells of the central nervous system, the result is multiple sclerosis. If it happens to cells in the connective tissue in the joints, the result is rheumatoid arthritis.

> • CARLOTTA: *I used to raise show dogs and work as a dog groomer. I was five-foot-two and weighed 200 pounds. I started having a series of mysterious swellings in my joints that would come and go without any apparent cause. I saw a rheumatologist, who diagnosed me with lupus. He said my joints were under severe strain because of my weight, put me on cortisone and methytrexate to relieve my symptoms, and handed me a diet sheet that prescribed a low-calorie, low-fat regimen. I wasn't willing to live with the side effects of the drugs. And I have never lost weight on a low-calorie, low-fat diet. Usually I gain even when I eat only 600 calories a day.*
>
> *I kept getting worse. Soon I couldn't show my own dogs because I couldn't walk. I couldn't work as a groomer because I couldn't get down on my knees. I had days that I dropped everything I picked up, so I didn't dare pick up my new granddaughter. I couldn't turn the key to start the car.*

Several theories attempt to explain why the immune system can become intolerant of autoantigens and mistake them for invaders. One is that viruses or injuries can change the appearance of cells, making them appear foreign and stimulating the immune system to create antibodies to these damaged cells. Because these antibodies attack the body's own cells, they are called autoantibodies. A possible example of this phenomenon is the damaging effect that scarlet fever, a streptococcus infection, can have on cells of the kidneys, giving rise to a form of glomerulonephritis, an autoimmune disease that ultimately destroys the kidneys. In Type 1 (insulin-dependent) diabetes, the damage may be caused by a faulty gene that creates either defective insulin-secreting cells in the pancreas or flawed immune system cells that fail to recognize the pancreatic cells. In either case the result is the creation of autoantibodies that attack and destroy the pancreatic cells.

Other theories of autoimmunity exist, each with its own adherents and critics. All but one have this in common: The only solutions they consider possible involve drugs that bring with them their own problems—steroids, nonsteroidal anti-inflammatory drugs (NSAIDs), and drugs such as gold, methotrexate, and interferon. But there is another theory to examine, one for which there is a nonmedical solution. Although unproven, Dr. Loren Cordain's theory is based on ample evidence that a substance in certain foods can confuse the immune system, causing it to identify autoantigens as invaders.

The theory is that cereal grains—wheat, rye, barley, oats, corn, rice, sorghum, and millet—contain elements that mimic substances in the human body, and that when these elements get into the human bloodstream, an autoimmune reaction can occur. To understand how this could happen, let's analyze what cereal grains are and how they are processed by the body.

Cereal grains are grass seeds. The purpose of seeds is to carry on the species from one generation to the next. If that is to happen, seeds must be protected from predators—animals that would like to eat them. Evolution is the process of developing protective devices to ensure that species remain in existence. Individuals within a species that develop the best protective devices live long enough to reproduce; those that do not, die out. So the protective devices are passed on from generation to generation.

Among the protective devices developed in the cereal grains is one known as molecular mimicry. Molecular mimics are antinutrients, proteins with a cell structure strikingly similar to those in mammals, including human beings. The effect of this is to discourage animals from eating grains containing these proteins; few animals will eat their own kind. Grains also contain cellulose, which human beings cannot digest. This is why we must grind and cook grains if we are to get nourishment from them. Grinding and cooking breaks down the cellulose so that it passes through the digestive system, still indigestible, but providing fiber and roughage that aids in the elimination of waste material. But the cells that mimic ours remain intact.[1]

Under normal circumstances, food is broken down and its nutrients are absorbed in the small intestine. Its lining is constructed so that nothing can pass through to the bloodstream except the nutrients the body is able to use. But the antinutrients can damage the lining of the gut. Furthermore, a diet in which starches and sugars predominate tends to be hard to digest, and the small intestine can send undigested nutrients on to the colon, where digestive bacteria turn the starches and sugars into alcohols and gases.

With alcohols and gases roiling around in the colon, some of the largely liquid digestive slurry tends to get flushed back into the small intestine, where it can cause inflammation and weaken the tight bonds in the lining of the gut. This allows larger molecules to slip into the bloodstream.[2] Some of these molecules will be from partially digested plant proteins, called lectins. Lectins in the blood spell trouble. For one thing, they increase the blood's tendency to clot. For another, the immune system recognizes them as invaders and sets about attacking and destroying them.

Remember that lectins are the plant proteins designed by nature as a self-protective measure to mimic animal proteins and discourage predators from eating plant seeds. The immune cells, having learned to recognize the lectins and destroy them, begin attacking the cells of the body that the lectins mimic, destroying them too. There's a lectin in wheat with a string of amino acids (the building blocks of protein) that is nearly identical to the amino acid strings in the connective tissue lining the joints, and another that mimics proteins in the myelin sheath that insulates nerves. Some plant proteins resemble parts of the filtering mech-

1. Loren Cordain, "Cereal Grains: Humanity's Double-Edged Sword," *World Review of Nutrition and Dietetics* 84 (1999): 19–73.
2. Michael R. Eades and Mary Dan Eades, *The Protein Power Life Plan* (New York: Warner Books, 2000), p. 143.

anism in the kidneys, and some resemble the insulin-producing beta cells of the pancreas, the lining of the gut, and the retina of the eye.

There is as yet no scientific proof for this theory of molecular mimicry as a cause of autoimmune disease, but there is evidence to support its components, and nothing has yet disproved it. The existence of plant cells with amino acid chains that mimic those of human cells is a reality. The "leaky gut" that can result from intestinal inflammation is a well-known phenomenon.

There is geographical and historical evidence to support this theory as well. Start with the fact that there is scant evidence of autoimmune disease in the fossil remains of people who lived in preagricultural times. Then consider the fact that autoimmune disease is most common among people of northern European descent; its incidence decreases as you trace the migration of agriculture diagonally to the southeast, to the Middle East, where agriculture began. Evidently, evolution has seen to it that the longer people are exposed to grains (grass seeds) in their diet, the better able their immune cells become at differentiating between self and nonself molecules.[3] ("Longer" in evolutionary terms is measured in thousands of years, not in an individual's lifetime.)

Once immune cells begin recognizing an autoantigen as foreign to the body, what hope is there of blunting the autoimmune reaction? After all, you might eliminate from your diet the grains whose lectins started the autoimmune response in the first place, but you can hardly eliminate the body cells that those lectins mimic. The answer lies in a group of chemicals called eicosanoids and, ultimately, in reducing the amount of insulin in your bloodstream—in correcting insulin resistance, in other words.

Like hormones, eicosanoids are chemical messengers that exert an effect on body functions. Unlike hormones, which are secreted by specific glands and travel in the blood to the locations

3. Cordain, "Cereal Grains."

where they do their work, eicosanoids are produced and perform their function within the cells; exactly what they do depends on the type of cell that produced them. Lab tests can measure the levels of the various hormones. Eicosanoids decay or are destroyed by enzymes and disappear too quickly to be readily measured in blood tests. But the speed with which they disappear belies their importance to your health and well-being.

Eicosanoids are involved in a great number of bodily functions; among them are blood pressure, clotting, the breaking down of fats, fluid balance and swelling, uterine contractions during childbirth and menstruation, sexual potency in men, the cycle of sleeping and waking, the release of gastric acid, the expansion and dilation of blood vessels and the airways in the lungs, the signaling of pain, and—most important to this discussion—fever, inflammation, and the operation of the immune system.[4] Prostaglandins are one kind of eicosanoid. They and the other eicosanoids (leukotrienes and thromboxanes) can be considered "good" or "bad," according to how they behave. Good eicosanoids control the proliferation of cells that is cancer. Bad eicosanoids are implicated in osteoporosis.

But even the "bad" eicosanoids can be "good" if they are present in moderation. For example, "bad" eicosanoids are associated with venous thrombosis, the formation of blood clots in the veins, which can be dangerous, even fatal. But hemophilia, the condition in which blood fails to clot at all, leading to uncontrolled bleeding, is at least as likely to be fatal as thrombosis, so it is inaccurate to say that the clotting action of eicosanoids is a negative factor. Clearly, some "bad" eicosanoids are necessary. It's also necessary to prevent the formation of too many of them.

Eicosanoids result from the breakdown of arachidonic acid, a fatty acid that comes from unsaturated acids in plants, and from the fat in red meat, organ meats, and egg yolks. Some people are particularly sensitive to arachidonic acid. In them it can cause

4. Michael R. Eades and Mary Dan Eades, *Protein Power* (New York: Bantam Books, 1996).

chronic fatigue, poor sleep, grogginess upon waking, brittle hair and thin, brittle nails, constipation, dry skin, and minor skin rashes—all of which are also associated with thyroid dysfunction, suggesting that there may be a relationship between arachidonic acid and hypothyroidism.

The chemical building blocks for all eicosanoids, good and bad, come from the essential fatty acids (EFAs) found in dietary fat. You want a liberal supply of EFAs. And here's where insulin resistance comes in: Insulin plays a large role in stimulating the production of bad eicosanoids, particularly the prostaglandins that cause inflammation. Conversely, glucagon has the opposite effect; it promotes the production of good eicosanoids.

If you've been concerned about an autoimmune disease, you surely know that doctors use corticosteroids such as prednisone and, in less severe cases, nonsteroidal anti-inflammatory drugs (NSAIDs, pronounced "EN-saydz") such as ibuprofen (Advil), naproxen sodium (Alleve), and even aspirin to combat the autoimmune response. Corticosteroids work by inhibiting the formation of arachidonic acid, the precursor to the eicosanoids; NSAIDs work farther down the metabolic line by interfering with the synthesis of prostaglandins. Despite the fact that both classes of drugs inhibit the production of good eicosanoids as well as bad ones, they can bring wonderful relief to people suffering from some autoimmune diseases. But they can't help with those where the autoimmune reaction takes place in the brain, such as multiple sclerosis and myasthenia gravis, because they can't cross the blood-brain barrier. For that, you must turn to the fatty acids, which can act in the brain as well as in the body's other cells.

Now that you know that what you eat can have a potent effect on autoimmunity, you can begin to investigate which foods and food components to emphasize in your quest for relief from—or avoidance of—autoimmune disease. You have good reason to trim your intake of carbohydrates, because they stimulate your pancreas to produce insulin, which encourages the proliferation of inflammation-causing eicosanoids. You have good reason to increase your intake of proteins, because they stimulate your pancreas to produce glucagon, which has exactly the opposite effect. And you understand that fat, far from being the evil substance that Western society has been led to believe it is, contains the fatty acids that form the basis of hormones and eicosanoids necessary to our well-being.

However, just as there are good and bad eicosanoids, there are good and bad fats. Conventional wisdom, which is not wisdom at all in this case, would have you believe that cholesterol is the worst of the bad fats. It is not. Without cholesterol in your diet, your body would be unable to generate the sex hormones that make you who you are in the most fundamental sense. The fats you most want to avoid are known as trans fatty acids, or trans fats. They inhibit the action of the enzyme that promotes production of the good eicosanoids.

Trans fats do not occur naturally; they have to be manufactured. Trans fatty acids come about when hydrogen atoms are added to polyunsaturated fats. Polyunsaturated fats—corn oil, for example—are liquids. To make them solid, manufacturers put them through a process of partial hydrogenation, forcing hydrogen atoms into the molecules of oil under high pressure and temperature. This changes the fat molecules into something that never appears in nature, making them better able to pack together into a more solid substance. This is the process that turns corn oil into margarine, for example. Partially hydrogenated vegetable oils are used in baked goods and many other manufactured foods. You won't find food labels listing trans fats, but if you pick up ten food items at random in the supermarket, chances are good that the list of ingredients of at least five of them will list partially hydrogenated vegetable oil. Let the appearance of this ingredient be a warning to you that the food contained in the package will enhance whatever tendency you already have toward autoimmunity of one sort or another.

If you're interested in supplementing with fatty acids, two you should know about are gamma linolenic acid (GLA) and eicos-apentanoic acid (EPA). GLA is found in borage oil, evening primrose oil, and black currant oil, and in small amounts in oatmeal, which you will probably decide to forgo because of its high carbohydrate content. The richest food source of GLA is in breast milk. GLA helps in the production of good eicosanoids by suppressing the activity of the enzyme that holds back their production. EPA is easier to come by, and it not only inhibits that enzyme but also serves as one of the building blocks of good eicosanoids. It is plentiful in fatty fish—salmon, mackerel, tuna, and sardines. EPA capsules are also available. If you take EPA, be sure to store the capsules in the refrigerator.

Remember that autoimmune disease is associated with the overproduction of bad eicosanoids, and that autoimmune disease appears to interfere with the body's ability to manufacture fatty acids, in a vicious cycle that you can hope to stop by taking supplementary EPA.

·10·
CANCER

IN 1968 Sir Richard Doll published a book detailing the results of his study of the incidence of several kinds of cancers in different locales. He found a surprisingly wide variance in the prevalence of different cancers among the communities he studied. He concluded that variations in local diet accounted for the variations in types of cancers. Between 30 and 70 percent of cancers were related to food intake, he wrote.[1] The significance of this relationship has never received the public recognition it deserves. Perhaps because we all want to deny that what we eat can do us grave harm, the association between food and cancer remains largely unrecognized to this day, except for the reputed connection between high intake of dietary fat and certain kinds of cancer, most notably breast, prostate, and colorectal cancers.

There is a surprising link between insulin resistance and those same kinds of cancer. Like most people interested in nutrition and health, I'd accepted the common wisdom about the fat-cancer connection. I had come to this belief through my reading of health-related news reports and magazine articles, not scientific journals. Going back to the journal articles that stimulated some of these reports in the popular press taught me an important lesson that I want to share with you now.

1. R. Doll, C. Muir, and J. Waterhouse. *Cancer Incidence in Five Countries.* (New York: Springer-Verlag, 1968.)

The lesson is that sometimes the results of a study don't show what the news reports —or even the author of the studies—say they show. Here's an example.

A 1998 study[2] was widely quoted as saying that researchers had established the link between diets high in fat and the occurrence of prostate cancer. Since prostate cancer is the most commonly diagnosed cancer among American men and the second leading cause of cancer deaths, this information surely led large numbers of men to adopt a low-fat diet hoping to avoid this disease. Most protein foods carry fat with them, so a low-fat diet automatically means restricting proteins and emphasizing carbohydrates.

As it turns out, the paper didn't say that low fat intake alone could reduce the risk of prostate cancer; it said that low fat coupled with exercise may have that effect. But it said so in such a way that it was no surprise medical news reports emphasized the fat part to the near-total exclusion of exercise.

The study was paid for and conducted by the Pritikin Longevity Center in California, where restricting dietary fat to less than 10 percent of total caloric intake is taught with almost religious fervor. Participants in the study were twenty-seven obese men with an average body mass index of 35 percent fat. (Remember that a BMI of 25 or more is considered overweight; 30 or more is obese.) These men had presumably come to Pritikin for treatment because they had enough symptoms associated with obesity to motivate them to accept severe dietary restrictions. In other words, the study did not include people of average good health, only those who already felt themselves to be in some health danger.

At the beginning of the study and again at the end of three weeks, doctors measured participants' levels of sex-hormone-binding globulin (SHBG), a component of blood that regulates

2. C. N. Tymchuk, et al., "Effects of Diet and Exercise on Insulin, Sex Hormone-Binding Globulin, and Prostate-Specific Antigen," *Nutrition and Cancer* 31, no. 2 (1998): 127–31.

the amount of sex hormones available in the body. SHBG levels can be linked to prostate cancer in that when SHBG levels are low, the male sex hormone testosterone is high. And high testosterone is indeed linked to prostate cancer.

Researchers also measured blood levels of insulin, lipids, and prostate-specific antigen (PSA), a protein produced only by the prostate. Normally very little PSA escapes into the bloodstream. Elevated PSA levels usually indicate prostate trouble, although the problem may not be cancer. None of the subjects had abnormally high PSA levels to begin with, although three had PSA levels considered "slightly elevated."

Study subjects were fed a diet very low in fat and based almost entirely on complex carbohydrates. They were also put on an exercise regimen that consisted of thirty to forty-five minutes of walking every day and participation in a supervised exercise class. At the end of the three-week program, the researchers reported, the men's insulin, SHBG, lipid, and androgen levels were all lower. Those who had slightly elevated PSAs all showed a decrease. Thus, the chance of avoiding prostate cancer was improved in every participant.

This study (and others like it) does indeed demonstrate that a combination of low-fat diet and vigorous exercise improves insulin sensitivity and reduces risks of disease associated with insulin resistance. But does it prove that a low-fat diet by itself offers these benefits? Absolutely not. It is well known that exercise by itself reduces insulin resistance. It is quite possible that low fat intake had nothing to do with it, that exercise did it all. Some of the decrease in androgen was surely caused by increased sensitivity to insulin. We know that one of the hallmarks of polycystic ovarian syndrome, which is associated with insulin resistance, is increased androgen levels in women afflicted with PCOS. The restriction of dietary fat may have had something to do with the decrease in androgen; we know that cholesterol is essential in the manufacture of sex hormones. These men weren't getting any animal fat, and thus their cholesterol intake was severely lowered. The liver makes cholesterol when it's lacking in the diet, but the effect of sudden and severe restriction of cholesterol in the diet may have temporarily reduced the amount of sex hormones produced. Furthermore, it has been repeatedly demonstrated that even a ten-pound weight loss improves insulin sensitivity. Controlling the study subjects' caloric intake alone could have produced the weight loss, independent of the restriction on dietary fat.

Another flaw in this study's report consists of its reliance on another study. The authors credit this study with demonstrating that "in people who are insulin resistant a low-fat, high-complex-carbohydrate diet improves their insulin sensitivity and thus reduces insulin levels."[3] If you read the earlier paper, you will find it does nothing of the kind. Instead, it sets out the same low-fat diet and exercise regimen used on the obese men at the Pritikin Center and reports similar results in lowering insulin resistance, as well as the cardiovascular risk factors of hypertension and high blood fats.

Nothing in either of these studies demonstrates any benefit whatsoever from a low-fat diet by itself. To do that, the authors would have split the men into three groups, one getting a low-fat diet without exercise, one subjected to a rigorous exercise program without the low-fat diet, and one following the full regimen of low fat and vigorous exercise. Having failed to test all three approaches, the researchers did nothing but feed the low-fat diet myth. It is instructive to recall that the organization that funded this study makes its money by putting people on low-fat diets.

It would be interesting to know how these men have fared since being released from the Pritikin Center—whether their weight stayed down, whether their blood chemistry remained in the improved state documented at the end of the three weeks,

3. R. J. Barnard, et al., "Role of Diet and Exercise in the Management of Hyperinsulinemia and Associated Atherosclerotic Risk Factors," *American Journal of Cardiology* 69, no. 5 (1992): 440–44.

and whether any of them remained on the regimen after they went home.

PROSTATE CANCER

While it fails in its effort to convince us that a low-fat diet will help prevent prostate cancer, the Pritikin Center study does demonstrate the increased cancer risk presented by insulin resistance in relation to the production of the male hormones. Another way in which insulin resistance heightens the risk of cancer is in relation to the hormone insulin-like growth factor 1 (IGF-1), which is elevated in the blood of people with higher-than-normal insulin levels. In fact, one study done at the Harvard School of Public Health and McGill University, published in 1998, looked at blood samples drawn from 304 men, half of whom had been diagnosed with prostate cancer and half of whom had not. Researchers found that the men with the highest levels of IGF-1 had four times the risk of prostate cancer compared to those with the lowest levels.[4]

IGF-1 is one of several growth factors related to insulin that regulate cell division and growth. Insulin and its related growth factors have been found to accelerate cell growth and division in tumors. When the body's hormones are in proper balance, cells divide normally, the resulting new cells are just like the cells they came from, and the body's tissues are replaced and renewed without ill effect. But when a hormone interferes with cell growth, abnormal cell division can take place. Cancer is a disease of abnormal cell division.

BREAST CANCER

Insulin resistance is a risk factor not only for prostate cancer but also for breast cancer. Researchers who undertook the IGF-1 study in relation to prostate cancer did so because they wondered if previous findings concerning IGF-1 and breast cancer

4. *Science*, 279 (1998): 457.

held true for prostate cancer, too. And another breast cancer study reinforces the argument that claims made about the intake of dietary fat in relation to prostate cancer are erroneous. In 1999 a survey of nearly 2,000 women participating in the ongoing Nurses' Health Study found no effect on survival in women with breast cancer of a low-fat diet.[5]

The Nurses' Health Study, which has been going on since 1976, gathers health information from 120,000 women, all registered nurses. In this phase of the study, researchers looked at the cases of nearly 1,300 women who had been diagnosed with breast cancer between 1976 and 1990. They found the amount of fat in the diets of these women after they were diagnosed had no relationship to their risk of dying from the cancer. The researchers did, however, find a 35 percent lower risk of dying among women who ate the most protein. They detected no link between how much red meat a woman ate and the likelihood that she would die of breast cancer. In 1997 Dr. Paola Muti and a team of epidemiologists at the University of Buffalo found that insulin resistance increased fivefold the risk that a woman will die of breast cancer.[6]

COLORECTAL CANCER

The same University of Buffalo study was the first to show a link between insulin resistance and colon cancer death, particularly among women. The study monitored the medical records of 22,561 men and 18,495 women between the ages of forty-five and seventy-nine. After seven years fifteen women and forty-two men had died from colon cancer. For each cancer fatality, researchers selected four healthy members of the study population, matching for age, smoking habits, and geographic region, to compare with those who had died. Nearly 27 percent of the women who had died of colon cancer—almost ten times the

5. *Cancer* 86 (1999): 751–755, 825–834.
6. Paola Muti, M.D. Paper presented at the annual meeting of the Society for Epidemiological Research, Seattle, June 1997.

number of healthy controls—had the characteristics of insulin resistance. This means that insulin-resistant women are nearly ten times more likely to die of colon cancer than women who are not insulin resistant. For men the difference was much smaller. Insulin-resistant men were reported to be twice as likely as other men to succumb to colon cancer. Researchers theorized that in the women, high levels of male hormones associated with insulin resistance were responsible for the increased risk of death.

Scientists are also homing in on the association between carbohydrates and cancer. Until recently there had been no agreement as to whether or not eating a high-carbohydrate diet increased the risk of colon cancer. But results of a study announced in June 2000 showed that the digestible part of carbohydrates—as opposed to the fibrous, nondigestible part—has a role in causing colon cancer. The results are true for both men and women, but the two sexes seem to be vulnerable in different parts of the colon.[7]

Women who eat large amounts of digestible carbohydrates—including all the simple carbohydrates and those complex carbohydrates that contain little fiber—tend to develop their cancers at the beginning of the large intestine, while men are more likely to develop theirs in the rectum, at the end of the large intestine. The risk in women whose diet was high in nonfibrous carbohydrates was seven times greater than that in those whose consumption was lower. In men the difference was only twofold. In addition to pointing out the importance of a high-fiber, lower-carbohydrate diet, the study suggests that cancer screening tests in women and men should be conducted differently, with women routinely undergoing colonoscopy—inspection of the entire bowel—while the standard procedure of sigmoidoscopy—examining only the lowest one-third of the intestine in routine screenings—may be sufficient for most men.

7. Marilyn Borugian. Paper presented at the annual meeting of the Society for Epidemiological Research, Seattle, June 2000.

Still another link in the colon cancer chain comes from a study that looked at the role the glycemic index of carbohydrates plays in triggering abnormal cell division, the factor that causes cancers to grow. The glycemic index indicates the speed with which carbohydrates become glucose and enter the bloodstream (see chapter 12). The higher the glycemic index, the faster the food turns into glucose and hits the bloodstream, and the more insulin is required to keep the blood glucose level steady.

It makes sense that high-glycemic foods—bread, pasta, potatoes, sweets, and table sugar—would increase the risk of cancer, because those foods require more insulin, and insulin can trigger rapid growth of colon cells.[8]

8. *Science News* 157 (May 6, 2000): 298.

·11·
OTHER CONDITIONS

I N ADDITION to the diseases and disorders already discussed, other conditions in which the connection to insulin resistance is less clear seem to improve when people who have them adopt the low-carbohydrate way of eating. Three are discussed in this chapter.

OSTEOPOROSIS

Osteoporosis, or brittle bone disease, is a growing problem in our society for two reasons: our cultural obsession with thinness, particularly in women; and the low-fat diet craze that grips our society. (Isn't it interesting that low-carbohydrate eating is branded by the nutrition establishment as a fad diet, while low-fat diets are treated as sane and normal?)

Osteoporosis is a potentially crippling disorder that results from the body's decreased ability to build new bone tissue. Bones are made of a tough protein called collagen, solidified by calcium, phosphorous, and other minerals. We tend to think of our skeletons as static and unchanging, but in fact our bones are constantly being broken down and built up in a process known as remodeling. The sex hormones estrogen and testosterone play a vital role in this process. A complex interaction of hormones balances the activity of two types of bone cells. Osteoclasts break down bone, and osteoblasts build it up.

In youth, the emphasis is on building bone. These are the crucial years, because the more dense your bones become, the less you will be affected by what happens later. People reach their peak bone mass between the ages of twenty and thirty. Bones that are not of a healthy density by age thirty will never be so.

Unfortunately, our society's high premium on slenderness in women leads to dietary habits that promote bone loss and ultimately osteoporosis. The process begins around puberty, when the sex hormones become activated. The bones begin to become more solid and heavier, because good nutrition and normal hormone development promote the growth of dense, healthy bones. Dense bones are heavier than porous ones. But teenage girls, desperate to be thin, notice they are getting heavier, and they start dieting to lose weight. Some become so afraid to eat that they develop anorexia nervosa, which is devastating to bone development. Even those that don't become anorexic often make poor food choices, avoiding proteins and fats and giving up milk for diet soda, thereby depriving their bones of the underlying nourishment required for a healthy skeletal mass. Of particular importance in bone development, in addition to calcium, protein, and fat, are vitamins C and D. Both aid in the absorption of calcium; if you're deficient in those two vitamins, no amount of dietary or supplementary calcium will prevent osteoporosis in the later years. And obviously, the more dense your bones are when you reach the age at which sex hormone production starts to slack off, the more bone you will have to lose before osteoporosis sets in.

By about age forty, the system has come into nearly perfect balance, with bone loss stimulating bone buildup and vice versa. Then the emphasis starts moving in the other direction, with more bone being lost than replaced. Decreased bone density is called osteopenia. Untended, osteopenia progresses into osteoporosis. Men are less subject to osteoporosis because their bones are more dense to begin with. After age seventy-five men and women share equal risk of osteoporosis.[1]

The low-fat obsession also contributes to the increase in os-

1. National Institutes of Health, Osteoporosis and Related Bone Diseases—National Resource Center, "Osteoporosis in Men," www.osteo-org/r603men.html.

teopenia reported in the medical literature.[2] We need fat to contribute to the development of sex hormones, and sex hormones are essential to produce healthy bones. The results aren't all in yet, but the three estrogen hormones—estradiol, estrone, and estriol—appear to play a crucial role in preventing bone breakdown. Even after menopause, when the ovaries stop producing estrogen, they continue to produce the male hormone testosterone, which turns into estradiol, the most potent form of estrogen. Women whose ovaries are removed are usually advised to take synthetic estrogen to reduce the risk of osteoporosis.

Typically, bone loss is a slow process; on average, twenty-five years pass between the onset of osteopenia and manifestation of osteoporosis. Many people confuse osteoporosis with osteoarthritis and assume they don't have a bone loss problem until symptoms appear. By that time, osteoporosis is usually far advanced, and treatment is aimed at preventing things from getting worse. The first sign of osteoporosis is apt to be a broken bone. As it advances, breaks become increasingly common. People with advanced osteoporosis can break a wrist simply by picking up a glass of water. A sneeze can trigger the fracture of a vertebra. The disease severely lessens the quality of life for those who have it, causing them to cut back on activities because of pain and anxiety. In about one case in five, complications from a broken hip lead to death within a year.

If you are a woman over sixty or a man over seventy, or have had repeated bone fractures regardless of your age, you owe it to yourself to have a bone density test. This is a simple X-ray-like test that is entirely painless and takes only a few minutes. If the result shows osteopenia, then you know you must at least make modifications to your diet and increase your intake of calcium and vitamin D to slow down further bone loss.

Among risk factors for osteoporosis are smoking cigarettes, especially after menopause, and drinking coffee, although other

2. John Kanis, Review of "Osteoporosis: Diagnosis and Management," *Lancet* 351 (January 31 1998): 379–80.

caffeinated beverages, including tea and soft drinks, are not implicated in bone loss. The fatty acid known as omega-6 PUFA,
found in sunflower oil and commercial fast foods, is suspected of
slowing bone growth. The more salt you take in, the more calcium you need to stay level with bone formation. Low-protein
diets are especially risky where bone loss is concerned. There is a
suspicion, not yet confirmed when this was written, that high
levels of the stress hormone cortisol may contribute to lowered
bone density. One of the long-term effects of taking corticosteroids such as prednisone is a very high risk of significant calcium loss. The same is true for excessive doses (more than is
required) of thyroid hormone. Antacids that contain aluminum
also increase the risk of osteoporosis. If antacids are really necessary, one containing calcium is a better choice.

Exercise is important in slowing bone loss. It's never too late
to begin to exercise. High-impact exercise such as step aerobics is
appropriate for premenopausal women, but can increase the risk
of fracture for women past menopause. For them, low-impact
weight-bearing exercise such as walking can increase bone density by between 2 and 8 percent a year. Even moderate exercise,
as little as an hour a week, can reduce the risk of fracture.

Research is beginning to show that the statins, the same drugs
used to reduce serum cholesterol, appear to build bone mass.
The discovery was almost accidental: Research scientists at the
University of Texas Health Science Center, San Antonio, noticed
that drugs used to treat osteoporosis itself work on enzymes involved in producing cholesterol. They guessed the statin drugs,
which target the same enzymes, might have beneficial effects on
bones. Subsequently, researchers at Brigham and Women's Hospital, Boston, studied the medical records of 928 women past
sixty who had suffered a bone break linked to osteoporosis and
compared them with records of 2,747 women of the same age
who had not fractured a bone. They examined the women's
health insurance claims and pharmacy records for the year in
which the fractures occurred and for two previous years. They

found that, compared with women who had no statin prescriptions, those who had been treated with statins for at least a year were half as likely to break a bone. In another study reported, investigators at the University of California, San Francisco, looked at the medical records of 598 women past menopause who were taking a statin to lower their cholesterol. They found that the women on statins had a higher bone density at the hip and a lower rate of hip fractures than those who were not being treated with statins. Some experts are saying that statin drugs are likely to become the treatment of choice for people with osteoporosis. But statin drugs are not without their shortcomings. They can be hard on the liver, making the choice of whether to use them to treat osteoporosis a matter of analyzing the costs of using them against the anticipated benefits.

FIBROMYALGIA

About five people in one hundred have fibromyalgia (FM), a chronic condition involving pain all over the body, difficulty getting a decent night's sleep, and sometimes overwhelming fatigue. It occurs more commonly in women, but a growing number of men are being diagnosed with fibromyalgia. Experts at treating FM think it is not an autoimmune disease, and indeed the conventional treatments for autoimmunity, steroid drugs and NSAIDs, are of little or no benefit in relieving fibromyalgia's symptoms. It is not progressive—that is, it doesn't necessarily get worse over time—and it is not life threatening, although the suicide rate among people with FM is higher than the population in general. This, however, may be due to the fact that fibromyalgia so often goes undiagnosed, and people who have it are often stigmatized by their families and coworkers as chronic complainers and hypochondriacs.

Fibromyalgia's cause and cure are unknown. There is no laboratory test that can prove or disprove its existence in a patient. Many other ailments can come and go in a person with fibromyalgia. Problems such as irritable bowel syndrome, low back pain, painful or burning urination, chest pain not associated with heart trouble, and itching or a feeling that something is crawling under the skin are common. Strictly speaking, fibromyalgia is a syndrome, a collection of symptoms, rather than a disease. It is quite possible that the syndrome has more than one cause and that a single treatment or cure will never be found.

Fibromyalgia is characterized by an imbalance of certain brain chemicals. Most noteworthy are deficiencies in growth hormone, cortisol, and serotonin, and a surplus of substance P, the hormone that signals pain. Therefore, most experts consider it a disorder of the central nervous system. This hormone imbalance leads some observers to the belief that its primary cause has to do with faulty digestion of foodstuffs and poor assimilation of nutrients, since ultimately all of the chemicals in our bodies are derived from the food we eat. Leaky gut syndrome is considered a prime suspect by practitioners whose orientation is toward complementary, as opposed to strictly medical, modalities of treatment. Yeast overgrowth is also implicated in some cases. People who have overcome candidiasis often report a marked reduction in symptoms.

Many people with fibromyalgia are hypoglycemic, which suggests they are also insulin resistant. Cognitive dysfunction, which people with fibromyalgia refer to as "fibro-fog" may well be the same phenomenon that hypoglycemics call "brain fog."

Chronic fatigue syndrome (CFS), also known as chronic fatigue and immune deficiency syndrome (CFIDS), is similar to fibromyalgia in its symptoms. I use the term CFIDS because I think it more accurately describes the condition and the way in which it differs from fibromyalgia. Pain, fatigue, disturbed sleep, and cognitive dysfunction are common denominators between the two disorders. People with fibromyalgia usually mention pain first when they describe their syndrome; people with CFIDS almost invariably speak of overwhelming fatigue after even the smallest physical exertion. Fibromyalgia is usually at its worst first thing in the morning; as people begin to move around, their muscles loosen somewhat and the pain lessens. People with CFIDS grow worse as the day wears on. Many people with fibromyalgia find that gentle daily exercise brings significant relief; those with CFIDS typically experience a worsening of their symptoms after exercise. Most significant, however, is the presence of swollen lymph nodes in most people with CFIDS, a sign of underlying infection that is rarely seen in people with fibromyalgia.

One interesting theory about the muscle pain so prevalent in fibromyalgia is that it is caused by sleep deprivation. One of the earliest fibromyalgia-related experiments, at the University of Toronto in 1975, took a group of healthy university students, hooked them up at night to electroencephalograph (EEG) machines, which measure brain waves, and woke them every time they descended into deep sleep. After a few days, all of the subjects complained of muscle pain and showed signs of cognitive dysfunction. Fortunately, they all recovered when they were allowed to sleep normally. Certain cytokines (immune system cells) are elevated in people who are deprived of sleep for more than a couple of days. These are the same cytokines that appear in people undergoing chemotherapy in relation to cancer. Such people also experience muscular pain and cognitive dysfunction. It is said that these cytokines also interfere with the brain chemical acetylcholine, which has to do with thought processes. That would explain the appearance of these two symptoms both in people who are sleep deprived and in those who have fibromyalgia.

One of the more striking characteristics of people with both fibromyalgia and CFIDS is an unusually profound reaction to stress. An adrenaline surge triggered by anger or the sudden perception of danger can leave a person with either of these syndromes in extreme pain and physically exhausted for days. Prolonged physical or emotional stress may be the primary cause of fibromyalgia in some people. Illness in response to stress is more of an effect than a cause in most.

Medical intervention in the form of pain relievers and sleep aids are called for when a person with fibromyalgia is in crisis, that is, when functioning is severely impaired because of pain and dysfunctional sleep. Most of the time, however, careful attention to lifestyle matters goes a long way toward restoring the person with fibromyalgia to reasonably good health.

Many experts believe that sleep disturbance has a great deal to do with fibromyalgia pain, so good sleep hygiene seems a worthwhile place to start. This means measures such as establishing a regular time to go to bed each night and get out of bed each morning, winding down before sleep time, and blocking out as much light and sound as possible. Quite a few people have found their sleep greatly improved by the low-carbohydrate way of eating. Almost invariably, those people report their pain is significantly lessened as well.

It's clear that hypoglycemia is involved in many cases of disturbed sleep, so it's no surprise that low-carb eating should improve sleep. Another factor that improves sleep and that also goes along with the low-carb way of life is daily exercise. In the case of fibromyalgia, this exercise should be started at a very gentle, low activity level—a few minutes of walking on a treadmill or level ground, for example—and increased a minute or two at a time when what you're already doing feels easy. Exercise improves mood as well as it decreases insulin resistance and hypoglycemia.

The fatigue that comes with fibromyalgia—and even more so with chronic fatigue syndrome—can often be relieved by minimizing the intake of carbohydrates. Rounding out the regimen that most people find helpful in managing both fibromyalgia and chronic fatigue syndrome is a program of determined stress management. Since unmanaged stress contributes both to pain and to insulin resistance, practices such as meditation or breathing exercises are quite helpful in dealing with these vexing conditions.

• *HONEY: I have had symptoms of fibromyalgia for at least two years. I have sixteen of the eighteen tender points, but I have not been disabled and have continued to work full-time. However, it took every ounce of energy I could muster to go to work. I'd come home at night, make dinner, and go straight off to bed for another sleepless night.*

In January 2000 I picked up Dr. Atkins' New Diet Revolution. *I saw myself in this book. I don't recall that he mentioned fibromyalgia, but many other things were very definitely me. I started the diet the next day. Within the first two weeks I started feeling so much better it was amazing. I was sleeping better, therefore the rest of the day was better. I found I had enough energy to cook better meals and to start thinking about doing other things, rather than just going to bed after dinner.*

I now feel lucky that I have also found a true path to better health. For the last four months on this program, I've had a chance to feel almost normal once again.

GALLSTONES

Cholelithiasis is the presence of stones in the gallbladder. The gallbladder's job is to store bile made by the liver until it is needed to break down fats. When our ancestors hunted for their food, they might go for days without eating, then consume huge quantities of meat after a kill. The gallbladder's ability to store bile was valuable. Today we rarely skip even one meal, and bile storage is unnecessary.

Eating a low-fat diet compounds the problem, since bile's function is to break down fat. When bile accumulates in the gallbladder for too long, stones are apt to form. These stones can be as small as a grain of sand or as large as a golf ball. Stones of varying sizes in one individual's gallbladder are common. Sometimes these stones cause no symptoms at all and are only discovered in the course of some other diagnostic procedure. Other times gallstones can block the normal flow of bile, causing damage to the gallbladder, liver, or pancreas that can be severe or even fatal.

When they cause symptoms at all, they are responsible for severe pain in the upper abdomen or between the shoulder blades. Between 8 and 10 percent of the U.S. population has gallstones. The tendency to develop gallstones increases with age. Women between thirty and sixty are twice as likely as men to develop gallstones.

Most gallstones are made of cholesterol; about 20 percent are made of bilirubin, a component of bile. It's the cholesterol form of stones that concerns us here, because the same insulin that deposits excess cholesterol in your bloodstream can also deposit it in your gallbladder. Also, obesity is a major risk factor for developing gallstones, partly because abdominal fat interferes with the movement of the gallbladder in emptying itself, and also because obese people tend to move less than those who are lean. Lack of gallbladder mobility causes bile to stagnate and cholesterol molecules to stick together. Heredity also plays a major role in deciding whether you will develop gallstones. Certain ethnic groups, including Native Americans and Mexican Americans of all ages, are particularly susceptible to gallstones. Among the Pima Indians of Arizona, 70 percent of women have gallstones by the time they reach age thirty.

People with diabetes and those with high levels of triglycerides are far more likely than others to develop gallstones. Interestingly, drugs that lower cholesterol levels in blood increase the amount of cholesterol secreted in bile, stimulating the development of gallstones.

Rapid weight loss is a major risk factor with gallstones. As the body breaks down fat during rapid weight loss, the liver secretes extra cholesterol into the bile, promoting the formation of gallstones in gallbladders that are infrequently emptied. Some people find that taking lecithin capsules helps dissolve the extra fat and prevents this from happening.

About 500,000 people each year undergo gallbladder surgery. The entire gallbladder, not just the stones, is removed. Most such surgeries are done with a laparoscope, requiring only a tiny incision and allowing faster recovery than open abdominal surgery. Only about 5 percent of cases are done abdominally. Most people who lose their gallbladders this way do quite well without them. Occasionally, when a person's condition doesn't allow for anesthesia, cholesterol stones are dissolved using drugs made from bile acids. However, the stones return in about half of all cases.[3]

3. NIH Publication no. 99–2897, January 1999.

Part III

LIFESTYLE CHANGES THAT COMBAT INSULIN RESISTANCE

As any farmer knows, the way to get the best price for livestock is to feed the animals large quantities of whole grains. Meat animals are sold by the pound, so the fatter the animal, the more money the farmer gets for it at auction. Conversely, when farmers want to raise animals to satisfy the market's demand for lean meat, they provide a high-protein diet. For those of us who have trouble controlling our weight, there is a lesson here.

Whether or not being overweight is a problem for you, now that you understand more fully the intimate relationship between the way you eat and how you feel, it's time to explore what you can do to achieve the best possible state of health. There's no way around it: if you're not satisfied with your current condition, something needs to change. This section will tell you what to change and how to go about adopting a low-carbohydrate lifestyle. It will also present scientific evidence debunking the myths associated with a diet that emphasizes proteins and fats.

·12·

GETTING STARTED WITH LOW-CARB EATING AND EXERCISE

I F YOU BELIEVE in the value of a high-protein, low-carbohy-drate diet but are reluctant to plunge into it, this chapter suggests a way to test your response to lowered carbohydrate intake before you commit yourself fully.

First, just to remind you how you will be flying in the face of conventional wisdom, as expressed by the nutrition establishment in the United States, here is an excerpt from the American Dietetic Association's *Complete Food and Nutrition Guide,*[1] with rebuttals based on scientific evidence and the experience of thousands who have thrived after they changed their way of eating.

A high-protein diet doesn't build muscle and burn fat as some people think. Only regular physical activity and training builds muscle strength.

This is true, but beside the point. No one who advocates a high-protein diet claims it builds muscle. As to burning fat, if your body doesn't have glucose to burn for energy, it will burn fat. Your body doesn't care which fuel it uses, as long as it has fuel for energy.

---

1. American Dietetic Association's *Complete Food and Nutrition Guide,* http://www.eatright.org/news/index.html#High.

While athletes may need slightly higher levels of protein, diets that focus on protein-rich foods, such as meat, poultry, fish, eggs and dairy foods, may be missing nutrients from fruits, vegetables, and grain products.

There is no documented need for carbohydrates in the diet. Proteins are essential to build and replace tissues. Fats are required for cell integrity and the production of hormones. As long as you have protein and fat in your diet, you can safely minimize carbohydrates. And no one is recommending that you give up carbohydrates entirely, anyway.

Depending on the protein sources chosen, the diet may also be high in fat and calories since fat contains twice the calories per gram as protein and carbohydrate.

Actually, more than twice the calories. Proteins and carbohydrates provide four calories per gram. Fat provides nine calories per gram. The fact is, though, that a diet rich in fat is self-limiting. You won't need or want to eat as much. Your caloric intake will probably be lower than it is on a high-carbohydrate diet.

Very-high-protein diets also can put a strain on the liver and kidneys.

There is no scientific evidence to back up this statement. It is true that people with damaged kidneys should not undertake a high-protein diet. But there is no logic in connecting that fact with the effect of protein on healthy livers and kidneys.

For those who do lose [weight], rapid weight loss may be water loss, not body fat.

The initial great weight loss is mainly water weight. Carbohydrates cause the cells to retain water. But after the first couple of days of low-carbohydrate eating, the major water loss is over and the rest of the weight loss is body fat.

This diet plan isn't a healthy eating plan for life-long health!

No comment is necessary. This is opinion, with no facts to back it up.

Indeed, many experiments have been done to assess the effect on various systems in the human body of restricting carbohydrates and increasing the amount of proteins and fats consumed. None has shown this way of eating to be harmful to people in normal health. Many have shown it to improve the various risk factors for heart attack and stroke. For example, a 1991 study done by the U.S. Navy switched ten healthy men, ages nineteen to forty-one, from a standard diet consisting of 50 percent of calories from carbohydrate, 35 percent from fat, and 15 percent from protein to a low (7 percent to 9 percent)-carbohydrate diet that obtained 73 percent to 75 percent of calories from fat and the rest protein—a higher amount of fat calories than most low-carbohydrate diets recommend. If those who say that dietary fat increases health risks are correct, these men should have been in direst danger. But they were not. Instead, according to the study report, their blood tests showed "markedly lower insulin, glucose, and triglyceride concentrations from consuming the LCD" (low-carbohydrate diet). Furthermore, the study subjects' insulin-to-glucagon ratio was lower, HDL cholesterol was higher, and other blood components improved as well.[2]

Even more compelling was a 1999 report to the annual meeting of the Endocrine Society by Dr. James Hays, who had placed 157 men and women with Type 2 diabetes on an 1,800 calorie

2. C. G. Gray, O. G. Kolterman, and D. C. Cutler, "The Effects of a Three-week Adaptation to a Low Carbohydrate/High Fat Diet on Metabolism and Cognitive Performance," (1991), http://mac088.nhrc.navy.mil/Pubs/Abstract/90/20.html.

diet in which 50 percent of their calories came from fat, 20 percent from carbohydrates, and 30 percent from protein. (This equals 100 grams of fat, 90 grams of carbohydrate, and 135 grams of protein daily.) For a year before going on this low-carbohydrate diet, the participants had been required to follow the conventional 60 percent carbohydrate, 30 percent fat diet recommended by the American Diabetes Association. At the end of the low-carbohydrate year, 90 percent of the participants met the association's targets for blood sugar, HDL and LDL cholesterol, and triglycerides. None had achieved this on the prescribed high-carbohydrate diabetes diet.[3]

Another 1999 report looked at the health histories and dietary intake of nearly 81,000 women and found that those who ate the most protein had the least risk of heart disease. It didn't matter whether their protein came from animal or vegetable sources, nor whether they consumed large quantities of fat or not. This study concludes with the words, "Our data do not support the hypothesis that a high protein intake increases the risk of ischemic heart disease. In contrast, our findings suggest that replacing carbohydrates with protein may be associated with a lower risk of ischemic heart disease." Then, perhaps to ward off the wrath of the low-fat fetishists, the authors warn, "Because a high dietary protein intake is often accompanied by increases in saturated fat and cholesterol intakes, application of these findings to public dietary advice should be cautious."[4] Even though they didn't find any added risk from fats, they issued what has become a standard disclaimer to avoid being attacked for departing from the orthodox view on animal fats in the diet.

You'll read about studies of the Atkins diet, the one that advocates the highest fat and lowest carbohydrate intake of all the low-carbohydrate diets, in chapter 15. Different diet books take

---

3. James Hays, M.D., speaking at the Endocrine Society's annual meeting in San Diego, California, June 15, 1999.
4. Frank B. Hu et al. "Dietary Protein and Risk of Ischemic Heart Disease in Women," *American Journal of Clinical Nutrition* 70 (1999): 221–27.

slightly different approaches to the balance between macronutrients (proteins, carbohydrates, and fats), as well as to other as-
pects of low-carbohydrate living. By the time you come to the
end of that chapter, you should have a good idea of which one
will best suit your needs and preferences.

WHAT TO EXPECT

You may be wondering what it will be like to make such a dramatic
change in your way of eating. Here's what I've learned, both from
my own experience and from listening to hundreds of others who
have made the switch. Your experience will be unique, because
you are unique, but it will follow a fairly predictable pattern. The
way your body responds will be influenced by

1. how high in carbohydrates, particularly sugars, your diet
   is now;
2. whether yeast overgrowth is part of your problem and, if
   it is, how extensive it is;
3. what your health status is now;
4. how often you eat in restaurants as opposed to at home;
5. who prepares your meals when you eat at home; and
6. how much support and/or resistance you receive from
   those around you.

If you are eating the typical American diet, breakfast is almost
entirely carbohydrates—cereal, a bagel or toast, or, if you're in a
hurry, a couple of doughnuts and coffee. You're famished and
sleepy by midmorning, so you grab some fruit juice and perhaps
some crackers. Lunch is a sandwich, perhaps with a couple of
slices of lunch meat, potato chips, a piece of fruit, and a few
cookies. You're hungry again in the middle of the afternoon, so
you have a candy bar and a diet soda. Dinner consists of some
kind of meat or fish, a potato, and a vegetable, maybe corn or
peas or both. Dinner wouldn't be complete without dessert.
Tonight it's a piece of pie. You had a tough day, so you add a

scoop of ice cream. When you head off to the living room to watch television, you bring with you a bag of chips and a diet soda. Hunger drives you to eat five or six times a day. You require a constant supply of caffeine to keep you alert. Throughout a twenty-four-hour period, carbohydrates make up 55 to 60 percent of your food, fats 30 percent, and protein the remaining 10 to 15 percent.

And if you've bought into the low-fat obsession, you're probably eating even more carbohydrates than that. Low-fat processed foods are invariably high in carbohydrates, particularly sugars. They have to be, or nobody would eat them. Next time you're in the supermarket, pick up a bottle of regular salad dressing and the low-fat version of the same kind of dressing. Read the list of ingredients on each and see how many more times sugars appear on the label of the low-fat dressing. Anything that ends in *-ose* is a sugar—sucrose, dextrose, and high fructose corn syrup are all forms of sugar. Now read the nutrition facts label and look at the amount of carbohydrate in a standard serving of each kind of dressing. Then go to the dairy section and pick up a quart of whole milk and a quart of low-fat 1 percent milk. (You could do the same with cottage cheese or sour cream.) Compare the number of carbohydrates in each. You'll quickly see how the carbohydrates pile up when manufacturers remove fat.

The first few days on a low-carbohydrate diet, you may find that you feel tired much of the time. There is a reason for this: your body is accustomed to burning carbohydrates for energy, and you're not giving it as much to burn as it's used to receiving. After a few days your system will learn to use fat for energy, and then you'll be amazed at how much more energetic you feel. If you start the new way of eating on a Friday (assuming your workweek is the traditional Monday through Friday cycle), by Monday you should be back to the energy level to which you're accustomed. Your energy level will eventually increase.

If you've been plagued by cravings for sweets and starches, those cravings may continue for a few days, but if you eat enough fat (and it's hard not to, if you're eating enough protein) your cravings will lessen and may disappear almost entirely within a week. I don't mean that you'll never again get the urge for a piece of cake or chocolate, but there's a difference between an urge and a craving.

Some people find that they become constipated on a low-carbohydrate diet. Some of these people misunderstand what constipation is, and are actually functioning well within normal limits. Most gastroenterologists consider as normal anything from three bowel movements a day to three a week, as long as the frequency is reasonably consistent for the individual. When your diet consists mainly of fats and proteins, stools become more dense and take up less space in the rectum. Therefore, there is less pressure to evacuate frequently. As long as your bowels move without straining and the stools are not hard and dry, less frequent bowel movements need not be a cause for concern. Constipation means difficult bowel movements, not infrequent ones.

If you do find yourself constipated, it may be because you are not drinking enough water. Everyone, regardless of the way they eat, should drink at least 2 quarts of water a day—that's eight 8-ounce glasses. Some people add another 8 ounces for every twenty-five pounds they are over their ideal weight. You excrete 8 ounces of urine for every 6 ounces of coffee you drink, so you need more water to make up the deficit.

Drinking this much water seems daunting at first, and it does mean more frequent trips to the bathroom, but it soon becomes habit, and the health benefits of being well hydrated are many. Allowing yourself to become dehydrated increases the risk of blood clots, decreases mental acuity, can cause muscle spasms, and strains the kidneys. People who hike in the desert, where dehydration can be fatal, quickly learn that if they wait until they're thirsty, they're already dehydrated. Here's an easy test: hold your hands in front of you, palms toward your face. If the pads on your fingertips are wrinkled, you're dehydrated. Fruit juice, loaded as it is with sugar, is not a satisfactory substitute for water.

If drinking additional water does not relieve your constipation, then you need to add more fiber to your diet. Since a low-carbohydrate diet is made up mainly of proteins and salad vegetables, your next step is to increase the amount of salad you eat. If you've gone as far as you can go in that direction without success, you should add a fiber source such as psyllium seed husks, which are ground fine and sold in bulk form that you can sprinkle on food. Psyllium is also the main ingredient in Metamucil and similar fiber products, but these are often sweetened to make them more palatable and can sabotage your efforts to reduce insulin resistance. Finally, there are psyllium husk capsules, which are more convenient than the bulk forms, but if you're going to get your psyllium that way, you must be religious about downing them with a full eight-ounce glass of water. If you don't, they will absorb water from your digestive tract and can choke you. And if psyllium doesn't produce stools that are easy to pass, there are over-the-counter stool softeners in pill or capsule form that you can try. It is very unlikely that you will get this far without success, however.

Notice I haven't mentioned laxatives. Most people can manage their digestive system's efficiency by dietary means and without chemical interference. But if you find yourself in discomfort and want a laxative, read the package label to make sure it comes from a vegetable source and does not contain a stimulant. Strong laxatives that include stimulants will invariably do more harm than good, making things move too fast, robbing your system of the minerals it normally absorbs in the large intestine, and causing a phenomenon known as rebound constipation. Many unfortunate people get themselves into an endless cycle of rebound constipation by using strong laxatives.

If yeast overgrowth is one of your problems, you may experience a few days of yeast die-off when you cut back drastically on carbohydrates. Deprived of their formerly rich supply of carbohydrates for nourishment, yeast will starve and die, leaving behind waste products that your body must work overtime to get rid of. Yeast die-off can cause feelings of nausea and malaise, and sometimes diarrhea. This is another reason to schedule your launch of a new way of eating until you have a couple of days ahead in which you can afford not to feel up to par. It's also another reason to drink plenty of water, to help your system carry off the wastes rapidly.

You may never experience an energy drain, constipation, or yeast die-off when you set out on a low-carbohydrate regimen. Not everyone does. Some soon find themselves amazed and gratified at their newfound energy. Eventually you will, too—if not immediately, then soon. And if the unpleasant symptoms are worse than you are willing or able to tolerate, then you can add back in a few more carbohydrates, continuing to avoid starches and sugars. Remember, though, that yeast can go into a dormant state and lie in your gut for years, waiting for you to resume your high-carbohydrate diet.

If you have an autoimmune disease such as arthritis or multiple sclerosis, there's no way of telling how soon you will experience a lessening of your symptoms, but most people in your situation do so when they eliminate grain-based foods from their diet. This is not to say you can realistically expect a cure, but in the majority of cases things stop getting worse. And in autoimmune diseases, that in itself is an improvement.

• *CARLOTTA: Back in the 1970s I tried a low-carbohydrate diet and lost a lot of weight. But back then I did what a lot of people did. After I lost the weight, I started eating the old way and gained it all back and more. This time I'm committed to low-carb eating as a way of life. I've lost some weight, but more important, my lupus has basically gone into remission. I have occasional flares, but not often.*

Last year I was able to finish and show two of my dogs. I can keep up with my granddaughter, who is now four. I still can't groom twenty dogs a day like I used to do, but I've started a new career in real estate sales, and I'm successful at that.

Many people find the most difficult part of low carbohydrate eating is dealing with the people around them, particularly whoever prepares the food at home.

> • SYLVIA: *In our house, my husband and I have a deal: whoever cooks doesn't have to clean up. He hates cleaning up, so he cooks. When I started the low-carbohydrate regimen, I told him what I needed in the way of menu changes. Our twice-weekly pasta nights had to end, and I wouldn't be eating potatoes or other starches, I explained. At first he thought his meal planning was going to become much more difficult, but I assured him I'd eat whatever main course, salad, and vegetables he put in front of me as long as starches were omitted. He soon saw how much better I looked, how much more energy I had, and how much better I was feeling. He decided to try the regimen himself and became a convert to the low-carbohydrate way of life.*

People who eat out much of the time often wonder if they can adjust to the low-carbohydrate way of eating. Fortunately, this has become much easier over the past few years. By the time you read this, low-carbohydrate eating will probably be even more commonplace and you should be able to expect any restaurant to be able to accommodate you.

> • RUTH: *When I began low-carbing, eating in restaurants posed a bit of a problem. Every menu seemed intent on "protecting" my heart by highlighting the low-fat "heart healthy" items. Those that didn't do that seemed determined to feed me fried foods with thick coatings of bread crumbs. If I was going out to eat with friends, I'd have to negotiate about what restaurant to pick. But I soon learned that steak houses don't mind dishing out a second order of the vegetable of the day instead of french fries or baked potato. I learned to order hamburgers and put the bun aside. I learned to ask the table server to leave out the croutons when I ordered Caesar salad with chicken. And today, with so*

many people adopting the low-carbohydrate way, most restaurants are ready for us. Recently, at a sandwich counter, I asked for a ham and cheese sandwich with lettuce, tomato, and mayonnaise and no bread. The counterman didn't skip a beat. At a university cafeteria I asked for the stir-fry without the rice, and the woman serving up the food put extra meat on my plate without being asked. What a difference two years had made.

Obtaining support from your family may pose a problem at first. There is often a theme in family relationships of not wanting anyone or anything to change, not even the way of eating of someone who clearly hasn't been well served by his or her diet in the past. The low-fat obsession has burrowed so deep in our collective psyche that you may find relatives looking at you with concern when you butter your vegetables or put dressing on your salad. However, those who mean you well will accept and understand your different approach to food when they see how your health and well-being improve. Until they do, there are other ways to find support.

•CINDY: *I haven't had a lot of support in this way of eating. At Thanksgiving, even though I didn't ask for any special treatment, my mother-in-law announced that she wasn't going to change the menu for the dietary needs of one individual. I handle friends and family by sticking to what I can eat, and I smile all the way to the bathroom scale. Most of my support comes from friends I've made on Internet e-mail lists and newsgroups [see appendix 3]. There's plenty of support out there if you look. It doesn't have to come from the people closest to you.*

Some people, in their enthusiasm, call attention to their way of eating and inspire criticism from those around them.

• ALAN: *I've observed that for some people, food is a religion. You don't want to interfere with someone's religion. Some people see how much I've lost, and they want to hear all about how I've done it. Others believe low-carb eating works, but don't see how they could incorporate it into their busy lives and don't want to hear how I did it. And then there are the food-as-religion people who ignore every word I say about it. These people can be spotted by about the fifth word, and it's easy enough just to shut up and let them live their lives.*

EASING YOUR WAY INTO THE LOW-CARB LIFESTYLE

It would be wrong to say there are no risks in switching from the typical Western diet to a low-carbohydrate lifestyle overnight. To go from 300–350 carbohydrate grams, the American Dietetic Association's recommendation, to fewer than 90 grams, the highest level advocated by any of the low-carbohydrate plans reviewed in chapter 15, requires a metabolic change that involves some degree of physiological stress. Some people can adjust without skipping a beat. For others the change is almost traumatic. I know of no way to estimate how your own body will handle the adjustment. If your physician is open-minded with regard to low-carbohydrate diets, you might want to discuss this with him or her.

To be sure, your body is well equipped to deal with stress. It must be, because you undergo some degree of stress no matter how much you try to avoid it. We tend to think of stress as being solely mental or emotional. You know you're under stress when you have a deadline impending for a job you've only just begun. But being too hot or too cold is also a stressor. Hunger creates stress. Loud noise does, too, and myriad other things that happen repeatedly throughout the day. Most of the time you adapt to the stimulus of stress without even noticing it. You adjust just as effortlessly if you decide on a sudden decrease in your carbohydrate intake, too.

But your body is accustomed to having an ample supply of carbohydrates for energy. If you cut back suddenly, increasing your consumption of fats at the same time, your system will learn to burn fats instead of carbohydrates as your primary energy source, but that doesn't happen overnight. Depending on your metabolism and past dietary habits, your body may think for a while that it's starving, a very definite stressor. In chapter 14 you'll read about the relationship between stress and insulin resistance, and you already know quite a bit about the problems associated with insulin resistance. There's one more thing you should know, especially if you're contemplating a major weight loss in this manner.

You can't change your diet this extensively without changing your blood chemistry as well. If you're insulin resistant, you most likely already have an increased tendency to form blood clots. Stress increases the flow of the adrenal hormones. One of the functions of these hormones is to increase the blood's ability to clot. A sudden large weight loss constitutes stress. So does a rapid change in blood chemistry. If you've ever had a problem with blood clotting, you should probably move gradually. In any case, you should weigh the risk of a blood clot against the health risks you live with today. To be sure, tens of thousands of people have gone low-carb overnight without ill effects. I know of no instance in which someone has died as a result of a sudden reduction in carbohydrate intake. Still, I feel I should call to your attention the risk associated with sudden added stress.

You can try moving into the low-carbohydrate range gradually by decreasing your carbohydrate intake by a certain percentage each day or week, and increasing your protein and fat consumption accordingly. This may not work if your insulin level is extremely high. In this case you'll probably be hungry and crave carbohydrates. But it's probably worth a try if you're not now driven by cravings. Start by keeping a food diary—not a bad idea in any case—for a week or so. Carry a pocket notebook with you, writing down every bit of food or drink that you put into your mouth. Include the name of the item and how much of it you ate or drank. If you can measure it, so much the better. But if measuring and weighing your food triggers the obsessive-compulsive aspect of your personality, an estimate is better than nothing.

For the next step you'll need a reference book on the nutritional composition of foods. For processed foods, you'll find what you need in the nutrition facts labels on the packages in which they are sold. Appendix 1 is a little tutorial on how to read these labels, what they tell you, and what they leave out. Also in the appendix are some suggested reference books, one of which analyzes common packaged foods and items sold in several fast food restaurant chains.

Next to each food item you have listed, enter the amount of energy (calories) it contains as well as the number of grams of each macronutrient—protein, carbohydrate, and fat. This information is found on the nutrition facts labels of processed foods and in the nutrition reference books. At the end of each day, add up the calories and grams of each macronutrient you've eaten. A sample food diary page appears in appendix 2. There you will also find instructions to calculate the nutritional makeup of your total daily intake of food. You can then decide by how much to adjust each macronutrient as you move toward less carbohydrate and more protein and, possibly, more fat, depending on how much of your diet is currently composed of fat.

That's one way to do it gradually. The other way is to learn about the glycemic index of foods and begin the period of adjustment by choosing low-glycemic foods as much as possible.

THE GLYCEMIC INDEX OF FOODS

The glycemic index (GI) ranks carbohydrate-containing foods on a scale from 0 to 100 or above according to the speed with which they get into the bloodstream and raise the level of glucose. Foods that rank high on the glycemic index cause blood sugar to soar. The result is a high output of insulin from the pancreas, resulting in increased insulin resistance and an increased risk of the illnesses that civilization has brought us.

The index was first proposed by Dr. David Jenkins, a professor of nutrition at the University of Toronto, in 1981 as a way to help people with diabetes determine which foods are likely to cause the least fluctuation in their blood sugar levels. As such, it is still the subject of considerable controversy within the diabetes establishment in the United States, although it has for years been an accepted part of diabetes management in Canada, Australia, New Zealand, and France. The argument against it in the United States is not that it is an inaccurate measure of the impact on the blood of starches and sugars but that it is confusing and difficult to use in making food choices. No authority seems to dispute that high-glycemic foods stimulate insulin secretion. The glycemic index appears to provide a good way for people contemplating a low-carbohydrate diet to ease their way into the regimen.

Jenkins and his associates fed healthy fasting volunteers sixty-two common foods, one at a time, in amounts sufficient to yield 50 grams of carbohydrate. He measured the effect on their blood glucose levels over the next two hours. He then compared this with the same people's response to an identical amount of carbohydrate in the form of 50 grams of glucose. By giving the study participants' response to pure glucose a value of 100, he was able to assign an index number to each of the foods tested. The higher the index number, the more rapid the rise in blood sugar.[5]

The effect of a low-glycemic-index diet on people with Type 2 diabetes has been tested repeatedly. In a 1992 study Dr. T. M. Wolever had people spend six weeks on a relatively low-glycemic diet with an average index of 58, and six weeks on a diet with an index of 86. These were not low-carbohydrate diets; in each case, carbohydrates made up 57 percent of total calories. Participants lost weight on both diets. Blood glucose control proved to be 8 percent better on the low GI diet, and total serum cholesterol was lower by 7 percent.[6]

5. D. J. Jenkins et al., "Glycemic Index of Foods: A Physiological Basis for Carbohydrate Exchange," *American Journal of Clinical Nutrition* 34, no. 3 (March 1981): 362–63.
6. T. M. Wolever et al., "Beneficial Effect of Low-Glycemic Index Diet in Overweight NIDDM Subjects," *Diabetes Care* 15, no. 4 (April 1992): 562–64.

In 1999 a research team at Hammersmith Hospital in London found that the glycemic index of foods is more closely related than dietary fat intake to the presence of HDL cholesterol (the good kind) in the blood.[7] High-GI foods not only stimulate insulin release but also trigger production of the stress hormones epinephrine and norepinephrine, which lower insulin sensitivity.[8]

Even more significant for our purposes is the finding that insulin secretions over a twenty-four-hour period were between 22 and 42 percent lower in people who had been on a low-glycemic-index diet for two weeks, as measured by urinary C-peptide, a by-product of insulin that indicates how much insulin has been produced by the pancreas. People who do not produce insulin produce no C-peptide. It is encouraging that even though the study participants' blood glucose shot up as expected when they were subjected to a standard glucose challenge test at the end of the two weeks, they did not show an increased insulin response.[9]

People differ in their glycemic response to foods. The GI is not an absolute measure, but it does give a fair idea of the relative impact various foods will have on your blood sugar level and therefore on the amount of insulin your pancreas will release in response to the food you eat. Since you probably won't eat only one food at a meal, the overall glycemic index of a mixed meal will be something like the average of the indexes of all the carbohydrates you eat. It's not necessary to worry about the total glycemic index of your meal, only to choose lower-GI foods to keep your insulin release in check. Proteins and fats have an effect on blood sugar levels and insulin secretion, too, but that effect is negligible compared to the effect of carbohydrates.

7. G. Frost et al. "Glycaemic Index as a Determinant of Serum HDL-cholesterol Concentration," *Lancet* 363 (March 27, 1999): 1045–48.

8. T. M. Wolever, "The Glycemic Index," *World Review of Nutrition and Dietetics* 62 (1990): 120–85.

9. D. J. Jenkins, "Metabolic Effects of a Low-Glycemic-Index Diet," *American Journal of Clinical Nutrition* 46, no. 6 (December 1987): 908–75.

What this suggests is that sticking to low-glycemic-index carbohydrates may be the ideal way to ease into a low-carbohydrate diet. You may want to lose weight, or you may not. You may need to reduce your blood fats, or you may not. You may need to lower your blood pressure, or you may not. But if you know you need to reduce insulin resistance and you're concerned about the effects of a radical change in your diet—going, for example, from the more than 300 grams of carbohydrates you're eating now to a carbohydrate intake of 90 grams or even less—you may want to try between two and six weeks on a low-GI diet before going to a very-low-carbohydrate regimen.

It is important to know that there are in fact two different glycemic indexes. Glucose is the basis for the original, developed by Jenkins. The GI of all foods is expressed as a percentage of glucose's 100. The other index is based on a one-ounce slice of white bread. White bread's GI is 70 on the glucose scale and 100 on the white bread scale. To convert the GI of any food on the white bread scale to the glucose GI, you multiply the white bread index by 1.43 (100 divided by 70, rounded up to two decimal places.) It doesn't matter which index you use, as long as you use it consistently. But if someone tells you the GI of a food, you need to know which index he or she is using. In this book, the glucose index is used consistently.

In the bibliography and in appendix 3 you will find references to books and articles that include glycemic index tables. Not all carbohydrate foods have been appraised for their glycemic index (can you imagine getting volunteers to eat enough celery to get 50 grams carbohydrate to find its glycemic index?), but this list will give you enough choices to combine with the proteins you normally eat so that you shouldn't feel deprived during your GI break-in period.

Generally, the glycemic index of foods is influenced by the size of the particles into which the food breaks down in your stomach. Small particles are absorbed and get to the bloodstream faster than large particles. For this reason, the longer you cook a food, the higher its glycemic index is likely to be. For example, the GI of instant rice nearly triples if it is cooked for six minutes. The more processing a food undergoes, including cooking in your own kitchen, the smaller its particles are apt to be. The less fiber a food contains, the higher its GI is likely to be. The same is true of fat. If you find yourself confronted with a food for which you cannot find the GI, and which you absolutely must eat, use these facts as guides to estimate the GI for yourself.

The table on the following page shows the glycemic index and carbohydrate count of some common foods, using glucose as the base. You will see that there is no relationship between the amount of carbohydrate in a food and its glycemic index. A good way to understand the significance of the glycemic index is to remember that foods with a high index number (70 or more) are fast-acting in terms of raising blood sugar, triggering the insulin response and providing energy. Those with low numbers (below 50) are slow-acting, and those in the middle (50–69) are intermediate.

Don't get the idea that just because a food has a low glycemic index, it is perfectly fine for you to eat and still get the benefits of a low-carbohydrate diet. Chocolate bars, because they are loaded with fat, are low-glycemic. But if carbohydrate cravings are a problem for you, you'll want to pass up the low-GI chocolate anyway. The food items listed were selected to help you get an idea of the variations caused by particle size, fat content, and processing, and to demonstrate that there is no relationship between GI and carbohydrate content. There is no intention to suggest that any of them belongs in a low-carbohydrate diet. If you choose to move to low-carbohydrate eating, you will be counting grams of carbohydrates rather than the glycemic index of foods. At the same time, if you become familiar with the glycemic index of low-carbohydrate foods, you will be even better equipped to make the choices that are in your best interest relative to your own personal health goals.

THE GLYCEMIC INDEX AND
CARBOHYDRATE CONTENT OF CERTAIN FOODS

Food	Glycemic index	Carbohydrate grams
	(glucose=100)	
White bread (1 oz)	70	15
Pumpernickel (1 oz)	41	15
French bread (1 oz)	95	14
Bagel (plain)	72	40
Dove dark chocolate (1.5 oz)	45	26
M&Ms (1.5 oz)	33	30
Snickers (1.4 oz)	41	17
Apple (medium size)	36	21
Banana (medium size)	53	27
Peach (medium)	28	10
Milk, whole (8 oz)	27	11.4
Milk, skim (8 oz)	32	11.9
Yogurt, low-fat with fruit (6 oz)	33	39
Ice cream, full fat, vanilla (4 oz)	61	21
Potato, medium, peeled, boiled	63	27
Potato, medium, baked, with skin	85	51

Source for glycemic index: Jennie Brand-Miller, et al., *The Glucose Revolution* (New York: Marlowe and Co., 1999). Source for carbohydrate counts: Corinne T. Netzer, *The Complete Book of Food Counts* (New York: Dell, 1997).

The fat content of a food item has a significant effect on its glycemic index. A bagel with cream cheese would have a lower glycemic index than a plain bagel, because the fat in the cream cheese would slow down the bagel's absorption, delaying its impact on the blood sugar level. Therefore, don't make the mistake of thinking you're on a low-carbohydrate diet just because you're checking the glycemic index of the foods you eat. If the low-carb way of eating is your destination, the glycemic index is merely a way station.

SUBSTITUTES FOR SUGAR

Nature gave us taste buds for sweetness for a reason. The sweet taste of colostrum, the precursor to breast milk, and of breast milk itself encourage the newborn baby to suck and thus to derive nourishment. Almost everyone likes to taste something sweet now and then, a fact that has been the downfall of many of us. Fortunately for people trying to combat insulin resistance, once you get sucrose out of your diet, your taste buds become much more sensitive to sweetness, and that taste is easier to come by.

Considerable controversy surrounds the use of sugar substitutes. Some experts say they have no place in a diet meant to reverse insulin resistance; others say they're acceptable; and some even encourage them. The dispute concerns whether sweetness itself can trigger the insulin response. I know of no study that has attempted to answer this question. My hunch is that some of us are conditioned to pump insulin when we taste something sweet, just as Pavlov's dog learned to salivate when it heard a bell, because it knew the bell would be followed by food.

I know of people who were unable to lose weight, and some who actually gained, on a low-carbohydrate diet that included liberal use of sugar substitutes. I also know of people who had the opposite experience. The consensus among exponents of low-carbohydrate eating is that given enough time, your weight should reach the level that is optimal for your health, which suggests that if your insulin is working properly and you need to lose weight, you will. I think you may find it necessary to experiment to find the answer that is right for you. If you're adopting low-carbohydrate eating to lose weight, and you can stand to live without anything sweet, consider yourself lucky and avoid sugar substitutes. If the thought of giving up everything sweet depresses you, practice moderation in using sugar substitutes. Then if you fail to lose, try going without sweet things and see if that makes the difference. Different sweeteners may have differing effects on you, too, so experimentation with a variety of types may be required.

Insulin spikes are not the only concern associated with some sweeteners. Saccharin was the first of the artificial sweeteners, developed in the mid-1800s. Sold under the brand name Sweet 'n Low, in the 1970s it was found to cause bladder cancer in laboratory animals. Canada banned it, but the United States did not, opting instead to put it on the Environmental Protection Agency's list of known cancer-causing substances. Manufacturers were required to place a cancer warning label on products containing the sweetener. In 2000 the EPA removed saccharin from the carcinogen list. As this is being written, it is not yet known whether the U.S. government will stop requiring the cancer warning label.

Arguably the most popular artificial sweetener is the nearly ubiquitous aspartame. Commonly sold under the brand name Equal or Nutra-Sweet, it is a chemical compound composed of the amino acids phenylalanine and aspartic acid. People with a metabolic disease known as phenylketonuria, characterized by the inability to break down phenylalanine, must avoid aspartame. Therefore manufacturers in the United States who use it in their products—and a great many do; if a product is advertised as "sugar free," it is likely to be sweetened with aspartame—must place a caution to phenylketonurics on the package label. There are no long-term studies on the use of aspartame, but it has been blamed by some for a variety of ailments, including headaches and neurological disorders. Some people find themselves craving diet sodas sweetened with aspartame.

None of the recipes in the back of this book uses saccharin or aspartame. My sweetener of choice is stevia, extracted from a leaf that is about 100 times as sweet as sugar. I know of nothing to suggest it is harmful (unless anything sweet tasting causes your insulin to surge). It is supplied as a liquid, to be added to foods a drop at a time. It can also be purchased in powder form, and in packets the size of sugar servings for use in coffee and tea, but I find a single packet much sweeter than a packet of sugar. Too much stevia leaves a bitter aftertaste, so using it requires experimentation. For reasons that are not clear, the U.S. Food and Drug Administration does not allow it to be marketed as a sweetener, although that is exactly what it is. It is labeled as a nutritional supplement and bears the advice, "May be mixed with water to dilute its sweetness." I mix it with lots of things besides water, as you will see when you look at the recipes.

A newcomer to the United States is sucralose, which has the brand name Splenda. It starts with a sugar molecule, removes three of its components, and replaces them with three chlorine molecules, making it hundreds of times sweeter than sugar. It provides no calories because the body doesn't recognize it as food. For the same reason, it has no effect on blood sugar. Unlike aspartame, which is destroyed by heat, sucralose can be used in prepared foods. As a tabletop sweetener it is just making its way into U.S. supermarkets as I write this. It has been used in Canada since 1991.

Another relatively new sweetener is acesulfame potassium, or ACE-K, which has been used in the United Kingdom since 1983 and in the United Stated in manufactured foods since 1988. It is beginning to appear as a tabletop sweetener under the brand name Sweet One. It is derived from acetoacetic acid (vinegar) and has a molecular structure similar to saccharin. It is about 200 times sweeter than sugar, but has no caloric value. It has not been tested for use by people with diabetes.

Aside from ACE-K, whose effect on blood sugar is not known, none of the sweeteners listed above is known to have any effect on blood sugar. That is not true for the sweeteners sorbitol, mannitol, and xylitol, which are often used in "sugar-free" products and which do elevate blood glucose levels. These three products may also cause diarrhea when even a normal quantity of a food containing them is consumed. They are not counted in the carbohydrate counts on food labels, but they are metabolized as sugar and contribute 4 calories per gram, just as carbohydrates do.[10]

One more sweetener you should be aware of is vegetable glycerine. It is barely sweet by itself, but acts synergistically with stevia, and perhaps with some of the other sweeteners discussed here, although I haven't tried glycerine with any of the others. It is particularly useful in situations where you can't add enough stevia to get the taste you want without that bitter aftertaste. Glycerine will allow you to use less stevia, and will enhance its sweetness but not its bitterness.

In appendix 3 you will find pointers to places where you can buy stevia and some of the other nonartificial sugar substitutes.

PROMOTING INSULIN SENSITIVITY THROUGH EXERCISE

Exercise is a superb way to increase the sensitivity of your cells to insulin and reverse insulin resistance. Put aside those thoughts about how you're too fat, or too tired, or too weak, or too busy to exercise and let me try to inspire you.

First there's the question of metabolism. If you're overweight, you probably know some small, wiry person who can put away twice what you eat and seem never to gain an ounce. "Life isn't fair," you tell yourself. "It's just my metabolism, and there's nothing I can do about it." That's partly true, but only partly. You're not likely to turn into a creature of all muscle and sinew, but there is a way to kick your metabolism into a higher gear, to get more energy and less fat out of what you eat. The way is to build more muscle by using the muscles you have.

Muscle burns energy at a rate much faster than fat. Every time you replace a fat cell with a muscle cell, you have added one more little pantry to use what you eat for what it's intended—storing

10. Maria Kalergis, Danièle Pacaud, and Jean-François Yale, "Attempts to Control the Glycemic Response to Carbohydrate in Diabetes Mellitus: Overview and Practical Implications." Canadian Journal of Diabetes Care 22, no. 1 (1998): 20–29.

energy, rather than building fat. The more muscle you have, the more calories you burn even while resting. Imagine being able to lose weight while you sleep. Is that enough of a motivator?

> • THOMAS: *My scale maxed out at 325 pounds, so I don't know exactly what I weighed when I changed my way of eating. When I started, I got rid of a lot of excess water, and that was very motivating. It gave me the incentive to go out and buy an inexpensive recumbent exercise bike. At first I could do about five minutes on it at very low speed, but I've been able to build up over time. Now I do at least forty minutes on that bike every day, at a rather high intensity.*
>
> *I can honestly say I haven't found the food part of this plan difficult at all. I'm never hungry. I eat foods I enjoy. In the last seven months I've "cheated" only a couple of times, and they were planned in light of a special event. Apart from that I've stuck with the low-carb way of eating faithfully. I generally keep my carbohydrate consumption between 10 and 16 grams per day.*
>
> *As of this morning I weigh 203 pounds. That's a loss of at least 122 pounds in less than seven months. With my current routine I lose an average of half a pound a day. The statistics that mean the most to me are that my pants size has dropped from a 54-inch waist to 36. My shirt has gone from a 19-inch neck to 16 inches, or from 2XL to M. I love buying size-medium shirts and they're a bit big.*
>
> *I feel great, physically. No more pains or physical problems. Even though I work out pretty strenuously every day, I'm never sore or feel bad. Right now I'm in better shape than I've ever been. I have a better profile than I did when I was in high school. I'm still not done, but I've built some good habits regarding diet and exercise, and I plan to continue for the rest of my life.*

As you exercise, your muscle and fat cells become more sensitive to insulin. Even simple aerobic exercise such as walking (it's aerobic because it makes you breathe more vigorously) provides the benefits you're looking for. It's easy to incorporate walking into your life. Look for opportunities to walk. Stop searching for the parking spot closest to the door you're going to enter. Before you get into the car, think about whether driving is absolutely necessary.

The benefits are quick to appear, too. In one study, five of eleven women were no longer insulin resistant after a week in which they exercised moderately by walking or cycling for an hour each day.[11] Both aerobic exercise such as walking and cycling and strength-training exercise such as lifting weights have been shown to have similar benefits, so you can choose the activity that suits you best.

The effect of exercise is cumulative; the benefits keep on adding up as long as you maintain your exercise program, however modest it may be. The more muscle tissue you have, the lower the fat component of your body. Prostaglandins aid in the synthesis of muscle protein. Muscular activity stimulates the creation of prostaglandins.[12]

There's more: If you succeed in overcoming your insulin resistance, you will be able to be less compulsive about avoiding carbohydrates. Remember the Pima Indians of Arizona, whose nearly universal obesity and diabetes was discussed in the introduction: Studies of their lifestyle found they rarely got more than two hours of physical exercise in a week. Meanwhile, south of the border with Mexico in a little town in the Sierra Madre mountains lives a small group of Mexican Pima Indians, close genetic relatives of the Arizona group. These people are uniformly thin. Yet their diet is higher in calories than their American cousins, consisting almost entirely of starchy foods—beans, potatoes, and corn tortillas. The difference? These people typically put in more than twenty hours a week of moderate to vigorous exercise, working to grow their food.

11. *Hypertension,* December 1997.
12. Michael Crawford and David Marsh, *Nutrition and Evolution.* (New Canaan, Conn.: Keats Publishing, 1995), p. 146.

CARBOHYDRATES YOU CAN EAT

Few of us can spend twenty hours a week exercising to combat insulin resistance and work off the effects of a starchy diet. That's why we may choose to focus on high-fiber, nonstarchy vegetables and low-sugar fruits as our carbohydrate choices. By doing this we minimize our bodies' demand for insulin and lower the cells' resistance to its effects. Luckily, there are many low-carbohydrate vegetables and fruits to enjoy.

Low-Carb Vegetables
Except where noted, a 3.5-ounce (100-gram) serving contains fewer than 5 grams of carbohydrate.

Alfalfa sprouts
Asparagus
Avocado
Bamboo sprouts
Bean sprouts
Beet greens
Bell pepper (sweet green)
Broccoli
Brussels sprouts
Cabbage (all kinds)
Carrot
Cauliflower
Celeriac (celery root, knob celery)
Celery
Collard greens
Cucumber
Dandelion greens
Eggplant
Endive
Escarole
Garlic (one clove)
Kale

Leek
Lettuce—all kinds
Mung bean sprouts
Mushroom
Mustard greens
Okra
Onion (1 oz.)
Radish
Red-leaf chicory (arugula)
Romaine (cos)
Shallot
Spaghetti squash
Spinach
Squashes—summer
String bean
Swiss chard
Tomato
Turnip greens
Watercress
Zucchini

Low-Carb Fruits

Even fruits that are relatively low in carbohydrates call forth insulin to handle the sugars they contain. Since one of the goals of low-carb eating is to require as little insulin as possible, fruit should be considered a special treat, reserved for days on which your carbohydrate intake is especially low. Fruit juices are always too high in sugars to fit with a low-carbohydrate way of eating. The following fruits contain fewer than 10 grams of carbohydrate in a half-cup serving, except where a different quantity is noted:

Apple (sliced)
Apricot (4 oz.)
Blackberry
Blueberry

Boysenberry
Cantaloupe
Cherry (sour, sweet, 10 medium)
Coconut meat (1 oz. or 1 cup shredded/grated, not packed)
Coconut milk
Currant (red, black, white)
Elderberry
Gooseberry
Grape (10 medium)
Honeydew melon
Kiwi fruit (1 medium)
Kumquat (1 medium)
Lemon/lime (2 inch diameter)
Lemon/lime juice (1 oz)
Mulberry
Orange (sections, without membrane)
Peach (1 med, 4 oz.)
Persimmon (American, Japanese, 1 medium)
Pineapple (1 oz)
Plum
Raspberry
Strawberry
Tangelo (1 medium)
Tangerine (1 medium)
Watermelon

·13·

KETOSIS, AND OTHER MYTHS ABOUT LOW-CARBOHYDRATE EATING

MUCH OF THE controversy surrounding low-carbohydrate diets concerns the possibility that you will enter a physical state known as *ketosis*. Ketosis is a condition in which the body uses fat, rather than glucose, as its primary energy source. Some experts say that ketosis is harmful. Others say it is the key to long-term weight loss and reduction in the primary risk factors for heart disease. The debate is reflected in the books discussed in chapter 15. Some low-carbohydrate diets deliberately court ketosis; others set the carbohydrate limit high enough to avoid it. This chapter provides you with the information you need to make up your own mind on this question. Your decision will be a key factor in choosing which eating plan to follow. Bear in mind when making that choice, however, that you may switch from one diet to another over time. Many people do.

If you have diabetes and depend on insulin, please discuss this ketosis section with your physician. There is a great difference between dietary ketosis and *diabetic ketoacidosis,* a life-threatening condition. I'll explain the difference shortly. You need to be sure that you and your physician address the difference so that you can monitor yourself for safety.

Your body, marvelously adaptable engine that it is, can derive its fuel for energy from three sources: protein, carbohydrate, and fat. Carbohydrate is converted into glucose for immediate use. It is also stored in the liver and muscle tissue as glycogen for future use. Protein is used mainly to build and replenish the body's tissues. It can also be converted to glucose in the liver, in a process known as gluconeogenesis (*neo* means new and *genesis* means making, so gluconeogenesis is the making of new glucose.) Fat is stored as triglycerides, mainly in adipose tissue—body fat—which can break down into glycerol and free fatty acids (FFA) to provide energy. Surplus carbohydrate is also stored as body fat, as we who are insulin resistant know to our chagrin. When fat cells are full, excess fat shows up as triglycerides in the bloodstream. The state of your metabolism determines the relative proportions in which these fuels are used. If carbohydrates are plentifully available, insulin will see to it that the glucose they provide is used first. If carbohydrates are scarce, the insulin/glucagon seesaw tips so that glucagon is dominant. Glucagon's preferred fuel is FFA.

To say that your body will burn glucose from carbohydrate first if it is available is not the same as saying that your body prefers burning glucose. Except for the brain and a few other tissues, your body has no preference. It will use either glucose or fat. When glucose stores are low, the liver breaks down FFA, producing a by-product known as ketone bodies, or ketones. Your brain cannot use FFA, but it will use ketones in addition to whatever glucose it can get. Some experts suggest that the main purpose of ketones is to provide fuel for the brain when glucose is scarce.[1] In a nondiabetic person, and in a diabetic whose blood sugar is properly controlled, ketones are always present. With a mainstream high-carbohydrate diet, insulin keeps the concentration of ketones to a level too small to measure.

When you eat few or no carbohydrate-containing foods, you use up your carbohydrate stores in about twenty-four hours. Then your liver begins the process of gluconeogenesis, using

1. Lyle McDonald, *The Ketogenic Diet.* (Kearney, Nebraska: Morris Publishing, 1998), p. 21.

protein to produce the glucose your brain requires. If you are eating enough protein, your liver will use some of it for this purpose. If you are fasting, your liver will begin using protein from muscle tissue to create glucose. Within another twenty-four hours or so it will look to fat for fuel, producing FFA and ketones. Ketones appear in the blood for transport to tissues where they provide energy. They also appear in the urine, where they can be measured using a disposable test strip, part of which changes color when it is dipped in a urine specimen or held in a stream of urine that contains measurable ketones. A diet that causes this shift in fuel use from glucose to fat is called a ketogenic diet. Ketosis is the metabolic state in which larger-than-usual amounts of ketones are produced. Glucagon allows it to happen; insulin prevents it.

Our hunter-gatherer ancestors were probably in ketosis most of the time, since they ate few carbohydrates until they adopted agriculture and began cultivating grains. Until we began eating cereal grains and starches, diabetes was unknown. For this reason, I find it hard to credit the statement that ketosis is a dangerous state in a reasonably healthy individual.

Diabetic ketoacidosis, however, is another matter entirely. Nondiabetics go into dietary ketosis when blood glucose is low. Insulin-dependent diabetics go into ketoacidosis when blood glucose is high, usually because they have been without insulin for too long or have used it up too fast, perhaps as a result of unaccustomed vigorous exercise. The concentration of ketones in the nondiabetic person in ketosis is considerably less than that of a diabetic person in ketoacidosis. If ketones accumulate in the nondiabetic in amounts that threaten to cross over into the range of ketoacidosis, the pancreas responds with a discharge of insulin, lowering blood ketone concentration to the point of safety once more. This feedback loop doesn't operate in a person with insulin-dependent diabetes, because his or her pancreas is not capable of producing insulin and therefore cannot counteract ketosis if it turns into ketoacidosis. If you take insulin, your doctor may want you to test your urine regularly as an extra safety measure.

> • GINGER: *My doctor says it's okay for me to be in ketosis even though I need insulin, as long as my ketone stick reading stays in the light zone. He's on the board of the American Diabetes Association, so I guess he knows what he's talking about. He says it's more important for me, as an obese diabetic, to get my weight under control than worry about fat or ketosis.*

Children who suffer from epileptic seizures that can't be controlled by medication are often put on a ketogenic diet. Unlike the ketogenic diets described in some of the books reviewed here, the epileptic ketogenic diet contains virtually zero carbohydrates, proof of the fact that the body has no absolute requirement for them. The main argument against the ketogenic diet for epileptic children is that it requires considerable work and careful measurement to prepare it. I have never heard anyone claim it is dangerous. It is difficult to understand why so many medical experts are horrified at the thought that some adults willingly put themselves into ketosis for reasons of health.

> • SYLVIA: *I've been in ketosis for more than two and a half years. For the first time in my life I have control over my weight. I have never felt as well as I feel these days. Every few days I monitor the level of my ketosis with a ketone dip stick that I buy at the drugstore. There's a patch on the stick that turns color along a scale from peach to dark purple. The darker the color, the more ketosis. I didn't lose weight any faster, and I don't feel any better or more energetic, if my stick turns purple, so I try to keep my reading at the lighter end of the scale. Ketone sticks show how much ketone you're dumping in your urine, not how much you're burning. I want to have a little more than I need to burn for energy, but not too much more. If my readings get into the dark end of the range, I add a few grams of carbohydrate or eat a bit less fat.*

GOUT, KIDNEY STONES, AND KIDNEY DAMAGE

Nothing is without risk. If you ride a bicycle or walk down a flight of stairs, you accept a slight risk of falling. If you are poorly coordinated, your risk of falling is increased. Similarly, if you undertake a diet low enough in carbohydrates to put you into ketosis, you run a slight risk of gout or kidney stones. If your heredity predisposes you to one or the other, then your risk is increased by a bit.

One of the products of protein metabolism is uric acid, a waste that is excreted through the kidneys. It is normally disposed of as soon as it is produced. Two things can cause it to build up in the bloodstream: an increase in production and a slowdown in its removal by the kidneys. If either happens, uric acid crystals can accumulate in the joints, causing gout, a painful disease also known as crystal arthritis. The ketogenic diet has been seen to cause an initial increase in uric acid levels in the blood for the first few weeks of the diet. But a small amount of carbohydrate can prevent this buildup. Five percent of your total daily caloric intake, which comes out to about 25 grams of carbohydrate in a 2,000-calorie diet, is sufficient. And studies of adults and epileptic children on a ketogenic diet showed a very low occurrence of gout, and then only in people who had a genetic predisposition to it.[2]

Similarly, there is little evidence of a relationship between kidney stones and a high protein or ketogenic diet. The exceptions are in individuals who have a family history of kidney stones, and even in those cases the problem could most likely have been avoided by drinking an adequate amount of water. Everyone, regardless of dietary habits, should drink two quarts of water a day. People on a ketogenic diet need at least that much. Aside from protecting your kidneys, there is another reason to drink water. One of the breakdown products of ketones is acetone, which gives your breath a fruity smell if you aren't sufficiently

2. McDonald, *Ketogenic Diet*, p. 77.

well hydrated. (Acetone, by the way, is why a diabetic who has fallen unconscious from ketoacidosis smells as though he or she is drunk.)

No studies of adults whose kidneys are healthy suggest that kidney damage results from ketosis or a high intake of protein. In fact, a study in Israel compared the efficiency of kidney filtering (the kidneys' primary function) in high-protein meat eaters and vegetarians eating very little protein and found no difference at all.[3] A reasonable precaution, if you are not sure how healthy your kidneys are, is to have a test measuring your kidney enzymes before changing the way you eat. It is true that people with advanced kidney disease should avoid protein, but to go from that fact to the statement that protein causes kidney damage is like saying that because you can't walk on a broken leg, it follows that walking breaks legs.

BONE LOSS

High-protein diets have been blamed for causing people to lose calcium, resulting in thinning bones. Some of the evidence for this comes from studies of children with epilepsy who were on the ketogenic diet, but in most cases those children were also taking drugs to treat their seizure disorder. It has not been shown that ketosis, and not the drugs, caused bone loss. The debate continues in nutritional circles, with contradictory articles in at least one case appearing in the same issue of a scientific journal devoted to nutrition. Aside from the epileptic ketogenic studies, most of the work that found increased calcium excretion in urine was done on athletes and bodybuilders who were supplementing their diets with manufactured protein supplements.[4] Protein from food is of a different chemical composition than

3. Richard K. Bernstein, M.D., *Dr. Bernstein's Diabetes Solution* (Boston: Little, Brown, 1997), p. 316.
4. U. S. Barzel and L. K. Massey, "Excess Dietary Protein Can Adversely Affect Bone," *Journal of Nutrition* 128 (1998): 1054–57; R. P. Heaney, "Excess Dietary Protein May Not Adversely Affect Bone," *Journal of Nutrition* 128 (1998): 1051–53.

protein powder. It is likely that other components of whole protein foods prevent calcium loss.

Other factors in the modern-day high-protein diet can lead to calcium depletion. Chief among them is the high intake of salt (sodium chloride) in most people's diets. When the kidneys excrete sodium, some calcium goes along with it. Excessive salt intake is commonly considered one of the leading risk factors for osteoporosis. It may be that those researchers who are finding calcium depletion in people eating high protein diets are failing to consider the salt intake of those individuals.

To be on the safe side, however, you may want to supplement with additional calcium and magnesium if you undertake a high protein diet. Current thinking is that men and premenopausal women should consume 1,200 mg of calcium per day, and women after menopause need 1,500 mg. Whether this comes from a pill or from food, or a combination of both, is an individual decision. People who don't do well with dairy products should definitely consider a calcium/magnesium combination pill. Since an adequate supply of vitamin D is required to make use of calcium, people who spend their days indoors and those who live in northern climates would do well to consider supplementary vitamin D. A dose of 200–400 IU is adequate (more in the darker months, less when sun is plentiful). Vitamin D is an oil-based vitamin, which means excesses are not excreted in the urine, as is true with the water-based C and B-complex vitamins. Oil-based vitamins can be stored in the liver, causing toxicity. The generally accepted toxic level of vitamin D is above 1,000 IU per day.

DIETARY FATS

It is virtually impossible to decrease your consumption of carbohydrates without increasing the amount of protein you eat. You are equally unlikely to increase your protein intake without taking in considerable additional fat. The first thing you will hear from those around you when you let on what changes you are making in your diet is an expression of horror. "But fat causes heart attacks. You'll kill yourself," people will say.

Dozens of papers exist that refute the contention that animal fats cause heart attacks. Studies have been done on populations all over the world, among animal eaters and vegetarians, and none has demonstrated a higher incidence of fatty arterial plaque in the carnivores. Still, the myth persists. Conspiracy theorists could have a field day with the fact that these studies have been suppressed, so the only information available to the general public is that animal fats kill us.

Instead of flogging cholesterol, let's look at the various kinds of dietary fats available to us and decide which will help us achieve optimal health and which will not. First we need to differentiate between three kinds of fats: structural fat, dietary fat, and body fat.

Structural fats are those that are used to build cells for body tissues such as muscles and brain tissue. The manufacture of hormones also requires structural fats. Body fat is stored energy. Triglycerides are body fats stored in cells. When they are so plentiful that they spill over into the bloodstream in large quantities, they give fats a bad name. High levels of serum triglycerides are a risk factor for heart attack. Body fat also provides the body with insulation to a great degree, but not always or entirely. If fat were the perfect insulator, obese people wouldn't mind the cold, but many do. Dietary fats can come from animals or plants. When they come from animals, they are a combination of structural fats and body fats.

Fats (also known as lipids) are made up of fatty acids, which can be classified as either *saturated* or *unsaturated*. These terms refer to the way the carbon and hydrogen atoms are arranged in the fat molecule. Animal fats for the most part are made up largely of saturated fatty acids. Their molecules are made up of long chains of carbon atoms, each attached to two hydrogen atoms with the carbon atoms at each end of the chain having an extra hydrogen atom. They are described as saturated because they have all the hydrogen atoms they could possibly have. They pack together easily, making them chemically and electrically stable. And because they cling together, they are solid at room temperature. Butter and lard are the saturated fats with which you are probably most familiar. They are the ones most commonly branded by the nutrition police as evil. Coconut and palm kernel oil also contain saturated fatty acids.

When one or more hydrogen atoms is missing from the fatty acid chain, the exposed portion of the carbon atom attracts a carbon atom from another chain, forming a double bond that is chemically and electrically less stable. A molecule that contains only one double bond is termed monounsaturated. Those with two or more double bonds are polyunsaturated. Monounsaturated fats are found in foods such as olives and olive oil, nuts, poultry fat, and avocados. They are reasonably stable fats and can be semisolid or liquid. Polyunsaturated fats, with their multiple double connections between carbon atoms, are liquid at room temperature and chemically and electrically unstable. They become rancid more quickly than saturated or monounsaturated fats. Because they oxidize rapidly (this is what causes them to become rancid), when polyunsaturated fats become part of a cell, they can cause damage to the cell. Damaged cells are potentially cancer cells. Antioxidants are our protection against the oxidation of polyunsaturated fats.

This is not to say that you should avoid polyunsaturated fats, however, only that you should be aware of their potential for instability and protect yourself from the effects of oxidation—and that you should avoid already oxidized (rancid) fats like the plague. Some polyunsaturated fats are essential to your health. While cholesterol, a saturated fat, gives structure to the membranes that surround the cells in your body, polyunsaturated fats give the cells suppleness and flexibility, which are virtues in a cell. To a great extent, your body is capable of transforming fats, both those we eat and those that are made from carbohydrates, into the fats we need.

DEPRESSION, CHRONIC ANGER, AND OTHER MOOD DISORDERS

Anyone who has ever used sweets or a special comfort food to combat the blues knows there is a relationship between what you eat and how you feel. But relatively little attention is given to the long-term link between diet and mood disorders. Evidence is mounting that what you eat—and what you don't—can have a profound effect on your mental health and emotional well-being.

We know that cholesterol is instrumental in making hormones, so it should come as no surprise that a blood cholesterol count that is too low can cause depression, hostility, or both. This information first came to light in the mid-1980s, when pharmaceutical companies were testing the so-called statin drugs that lower serum cholesterol. Researchers were puzzled to find that people taking the drugs started dying from causes that seemed to have nothing to do with elevated cholesterol. They were performing acts of violence and committing suicide at a surprisingly high rate. Since then, other reports have shown that people with unusually low cholesterol (usually counts below 140) are more likely than others to kill themselves. A 1995 study in the *American Journal of Psychiatry* divided the medical records of study subjects into four groups, according to their cholesterol levels. Researchers found that the men in the lowest quarter were twice as likely to have committed suicide.[5] Dr. Patricia Kane has reported a strong link between very low cholesterol and impulsive and aggressive behavior.[6]

5. J. A. Golier et al., "Low Serum Cholesterol Level and Attempted Suicide," *American Journal of Psychiatry* 152 (1995): 419–23.
6. Patricia Kane, "Understanding the Biochemical and Biobehavioral Nexus of Depression," *Explore!* 8, no. 1. (1997).

Depression may be the underlying cause of such behavior. Links between low total cholesterol (hypocholesterolemia) and depression have shown up in a half-dozen studies in the past few years. In one, researchers in Finland found that among 29,000 men, those with low total cholesterol were at greater risk of being hospitalized for major depression.[7]

The mechanism behind this is not yet understood. Some suggest that the lack of cholesterol reduces the production of the hormone serotonin, so well known to affect mood that the first thing many physicians do when they see a depressed patient is to write a prescription for a mood-altering drug such as Prozac or Zoloft. These drugs are believed to increase the amount of serotonin in the brain, although the mechanism by which they work is not well understood. Dr. Patricia Kane theorizes that a deficiency in blood fats in the brain allows immune system cells to cause inflammation, affecting mood and behavior in a negative way.[8]

The liver normally manufactures cholesterol on its own, with the aid of the hormone HMG CoA reductase, which is activated by insulin and switched off by glucagon. Even the most rigorous low-fat diet can lower serum cholesterol by only 20 percent. But in some people that 20 percent may mean the critical difference between a normal cholesterol count and too little cholesterol. It may also be true that some cases of hypocholesterolemia are masked by the way low-fat foods are loaded with sugar, which may raise serotonin levels above those that would trigger mood disturbances.

7. Peter Jaret, "Can Your Cholesterol Be Too Low?" Healtheon/WebMD, June 30, 2000, quoting *British Journal of Psychiatry*, September 1999.
8. Kane, "Nexus of Depression."

·14·
HIDDEN TRIGGERS
OF INSULIN RESISTANCE

IT'S PROBABLY impossible to list all the factors that can promote insulin resistance, or to eliminate every one of them
from our lives. But knowledge is power, and with that in mind,
you want to know as much as you can about environmental
and lifestyle changes that can help you promote insulin sensitivity. While the tendency toward insulin resistance is an inherited trait, there's no reason not to do everything you can to
combat it.

TOBACCO

Not only does tobacco increase the amount of free radicals circulating in your body, exposing your cells to the risk of cancer-
causing damage, but it also dramatically increases the level of
clot-building fibrinogen in your blood. And nicotine also increases insulin resistance by a mechanism that is not yet understood. A research team headed by Dr. F. S. Facchini showed that
the more you smoke, the more insulin resistant you become.[1]
There is reason to believe that ceasing to smoke reverses the
process. Unfortunately, smokers can't expect to see benefits of

1. F. S. Facchini et al., "Insulin Resistance and Cigarette Smoking," *Lancet* 339
(1992): 1128–30.

quitting as long as they use aids such as the nicotine patch or nicotine-containing chewing gum.[2]

This can be a can't-win situation: People tend to gain weight when they stop smoking, and weight gain is also associated with increasing insulin resistance. There are two ways to deal with this conundrum. You can stop smoking and start counting carbohydrates at the same time to minimize the likelihood that you will gain weight. Or, if that feels like too radical a change to take on all at once, stop smoking and accept the likelihood of weight gain, promising yourself that you'll get after the weight problem after you've got nicotine out of your system—in a month or six weeks, most likely. The second approach makes more sense if you choose to use nicotine gum or the patch to ease you through the withdrawal period.

> • *MARY: By the end of the day, my fingers and toes were numb. I didn't want to believe that smoking had anything to do with it, any more than I wanted to believe that my annual December bout with pneumonia was related to smoking. I decided to quit smoking only long enough to prove my theory that I had some disease of the nervous system. If I quit, and the day-end numbness continued, I'd be vindicated, so a certain amount of sheer cussedness went into my decision to quit—that and the fear of becoming an amputee like my uncle Bill. I put out my last cigarette at bedtime on the last Saturday night in July, 1969. If you know anything about addiction, you know that a true addict can tell you the date of his or her last smoke, drink, or drug hit. The next night there was no numbness. Part of my deal with myself was that if there was no numbness without nicotine, I'd quit for good. I won't pretend it was easy. It was pretty awful for the first three weeks.*

2. B. Eliasson, M. R. Taskinen, and U. Smith, "Long-Term Use of Nicotine Gum is Associated with Hyperinsulinemia and Insulin Resistance," *Circulation* 94 (1996): 878–81; A. R. Assali et al., "Weight Gain and Insulin Resistance during Nicotine Replacement Therapy," *Clinical Cardiology* 22 (1999): 357–60.

Here's a hint if you want to quit smoking: every time you get the craving, brush your teeth. Or, if that's not possible, pop a long-lasting mint into your mouth. The theory behind this suggestion is this: If you can occupy your mouth with something other than a cigarette for a couple of minutes, the craving will diminish for a while. And each time you succeed in resisting the urge, it will take a little longer to return. Also, you're less likely to crave a smoke when you have a fresh, clean taste in your mouth.

There is no question that smoking interferes with the action of insulin, forcing your pancreas to deliver still more insulin in the familiar pattern that leads to or increases insulin resistance.[3] Still to be determined is whether the interference comes from nicotine, carbon monoxide, or other agents in inhaled cigarette smoke. It is known, however, that nicotine mimics the action of the hormone epinephrine, and we know that epinephrine inhibits the action of insulin. Furthermore, at least one study has found increased insulin resistance in otherwise healthy men using the nicotine patch, which suggests that nicotine is the culprit and that smokeless tobacco or the patch are not the best ways to cure a smoking habit when insulin resistance is a factor.

CAFFEINE

If you doubt that caffeine is a drug, you've never drunk coffee and never seen a habitual coffee drinker searching for a cup, or else you're a caffeine addict yourself in deep denial. Caffeine has a potent effect on insulin resistance in two ways. First, insulin resistance raises blood sugar levels—which is why people needing a caffeine fix grow irritable and shaky, and why a caffeine-withdrawal headache is so common. Anything that raises blood sugar calls for an insulin surge, and you know what that leads to: insulin

3. Giovanni Targher et al., "Cigarette Smoking and Insulin Resistance in Patients with Noninsulin-Dependent Diabetes Mellitus," *Journal of Endocrinology and Metabolism* 82 (1997): 3619–24.

resistance. An experiment in which subjects were given a dose of caffeine equal to six cups of coffee produced in them a measurable degree of insulin resistance, comparable to that seen in Type 2 diabetes.[4] Second, caffeine raises stress hormone levels. People who drink coffee throughout the day walk around in a physiological state of chronic stress. As you will see shortly, chronic stress has been linked to the development of insulin resistance.[5]

- *MARY: I'm a former twelve-cup-a-day coffee drinker. And I don't mean twelve dainty little cups, either. For years I always had on my desk the largest coffee mug I could find. As soon as I emptied it, I hit the coffee machine for another dose. I refused to believe that caffeine could be interfering with my sleep. Want to know how good I was at denial? At one time in my life I insisted there was no connection between the fact that I was smoking three packs of cigarettes a day and that I came down with pneumonia every December.*

  When my husband and I sold our business, we wanted someone to take care of us for a while, so we headed for a health spa in Maine. It never occurred to me that there would be nothing with caffeine there. The headache I got from sudden caffeine withdrawal was amazing. It lasted four days, during which there was nothing in my world but pain. We were at the spa for another week. The headache was gone, and I had a fine time. I guess I was pretty well decaffeinated by the time we left, but I couldn't leave it alone. As soon as we got into the car I said to my husband, "Take me to McDonald's. I need a cup of coffee." After one cup, I think I could have flown home without an airplane, I was so high.

  I never went back to guzzling coffee the way I used to, but it was years before I decided to give it up once and for all. That time I tapered off, decreasing by half a cup at a time. I thought I'd never have enough energy to get through the day without my

4. Stephen Cherniske, *Caffeine Blues* (New York: Warner Books, 1998), p. 199.
5. K. Raikkonen, et al., "Psychosocial Stress and the Insulin Resistance Syndrome," *Metabolism* 45 (1996): 1533–38.

caffeine, but it hasn't turned out that way. I've tried decaf coffee a couple of times since then, and even that little bit of caffeine makes my heart pound and keeps me awake at night. I won't say I don't miss my coffee. I love the taste of the stuff. But I don't miss the physical problems that went along with it.

MEDICATIONS AND SUPPLEMENTS

It's one of those ironic paradoxes that some of the drugs used to treat hypertension are accused of increasing insulin resistance. Both beta blockers (which interfere with certain nerve endings that are stimulated by the adrenal stress hormones) and diuretics (which stimulate the removal of fluid from the body) have been blamed in separate studies by S. Jacob, G. Fragasso, and R. Reneland.[6] Still, if you have high blood pressure that requires medical treatment, it may well be that the risks of going untreated outweigh those of a beta blocker or diuretic. You might do well to ask that your doctor prescribe a vasodilating beta blocker or nonthiazide diuretic. Also, antihypertensive drugs classified as ACE inhibitors, alpha agonists, and calcium channel blockers have not been found to foster insulin resistance.

Glucosamine sulfate, a popular over-the-counter nutritional supplement, also has some effect on insulin resistance. Glucosamine has been shown to be beneficial in restoring cartilage in people with osteoarthritis and other chronic joint diseases. Scientists have commonly used glucosamine to induce diabetes in laboratory animals, but until recently no one thought it might do the same in human beings. Now it has been found to promote insulin resistance in an experiment with nondiabetic study subjects,

6. S. Jacob et al., "Beta-blocking Agents in Patients with Insulin Resistance: Effects of Vasodilating Beta-blockers," *Blood Pressure* 8, nos. 5–6 (1999): 261–68; G. Fragasso et al., "Differential Effects of Selective Beta-adrenergic Blockade on Insulin Sensitivity and Release in Control Subjects and in Patients with Angina and Normal Coronary Arteries (Syndrome X,)" *Italian Journal of Cardiology* 28, no. 6 (June 1998): 623–29; R. Reneland et al., "Induction of Insulin Resistance by Beta-blockade but not ACE-inhibition: Long-term Treatment with Atenolol or Trandolapril," *Journal of Human Hypertension* 14, no. 3 (2000): 175–80.

prompting the researchers to urge doctors to warn their diabetic patients to pay extra attention to monitoring their blood sugars.[7]

Glucosamine's effect on insulin resistance is not well understood. But it is known that low doses of glucosamine given intravenously cut in half the amount of glucose muscle cells take in. The strength of glucosamine's effect when it's taken in pill form depends on the body weight of the person taking it. In a person who weighs 150 pounds, a dose of 500 mg could have this effect. In general, the label on a bottle of glucosamine capsules recommends taking 1,500 mg each day.

If you have arthritis and are concerned that glucosamine may interfere with the health improvements you're trying to achieve, consider chondroitin, another dietary supplement that serves the same purpose as glucosamine. So far, it has not been implicated in relation to insulin resistance. You might want to ask your physician about it if you're currently taking glucosamine.

Some antidepressants exacerbate insulin resistance. Ironically, depression often accompanies insulin resistance, perhaps the result of the blood sugar roller-coaster insulin resistance produces in some people. Depression also may accompany insulin-resistance-related complications such as a heart attack. Often people who take prescribed antidepressants discover to their dismay that they cannot avoid gaining weight. The tricyclic antidepressants amitriptyline and nortriptyline are the two main culprits. A 1997 experiment using nortriptyline included diabetic patients with a diagnosis of clinical depression. Its goal was to see whether patients who were less depressed would have better control over their blood sugars. The result was that while the patients did a better job of complying with their diabetes control regimen, their blood sugars did not improve.[8]

7. Anthony Almada, research study presented at Experimental Biology 2000 conference, April 18, 2000, San Diego, California.
8. E. S. Paykel et al., "Amitriptyline, Weight Gain and Carbohydrate Craving: A Side Effect," *British Journal of Psychiatry* 123, no. 576 (November 1973): 501–507; P. J. Lustman et al., "Effects of Nortriptyline on Depression and Glycemic Control in Diabetes: Results of a Double-blind, Placebo-controlled Trial," *Psychosomatic Medicine* 59, no. 3 (May–June 1997): 241–50.

If you're already taking an antidepressant when you start a low-carbohydrate diet, you may find it harder to get the weight control results you are looking for. Don't blame yourself, don't give up, but do mention the problem to your physician. Interestingly, a 1992 study by Dr. B. J. Potter van Loon found that the antidepressant fluoxetine (brand name is Prozac) did not cause insulin resistance and may in fact have the opposite effect.[9] It lowers insulin resistance in both diabetic and nondiabetic individuals. Typically a person will lose five to eight pounds initially, but it doesn't cause weight loss in the long run.

As this was being written, psychiatrists were receiving notices that the mood-altering drugs Zyprexa (olanzapine) and Clozaril (closapine) were thought to cause diabetes in some overweight, insulin-resistant patients.

STRESS

A life without stress would be exceedingly boring—and boredom is a stressor in itself. There are physical stresses—hunger, cold, heat, and fatigue; psychological stressors—time pressure, things that make us angry or annoyed, uncertainties or unpleasantness at work and in personal relationships, traffic jams; and traumatic stresses—injury and pain. Somewhere between physical and psychological stressors are things we often can't avoid such as loud noises and noxious odors. Stress is an inevitable part of life. Telling you to avoid stress is about as helpful as telling you to avoid thinking. It can't be done. And when the doctor tells you that stress is causing your health problem, it probably feels like you're being blamed for your own condition, although the doctor may not mean that at all.

Let's draw a distinction between acute and chronic stress. Stress that occurs suddenly and is of short duration is acute

---

9. B. J. Potter van Loon et al., "Fluoxetine Increases Insulin Action in Obese Nondiabetic and in Obese Non-Insulin-Dependent Diabetic Individuals," *International Journal of Obesity and Related Metabolic Disorders* 16, no. 2 (February 1992): 79–85.

stress: you're driving to work in your car, and a child runs out in front of you. You swerve and miss the child, but your heart thumps in your chest for a few minutes after you've realized that the danger is over. That's acute stress. You have a deadline coming up at work for a report you've been working on for weeks. Some of the people you're depending on for information to use in the report haven't responded to your requests. You know you're going to be late. You've asked your boss for help in getting the information, but the help hasn't been forthcoming. Still, your boss holds you accountable for getting the report in on time. He needs it to make a presentation to his boss. When you get to your desk, there's a note asking you to call your boss the minute you get in. You've been under chronic stress for weeks over this report and the lack of support you've received. Now the stress becomes acute as well, as anger rises in you, and your heart starts pounding again.

When you're faced with a situation that causes acute stress, your body needs extra energy to respond. It's as though you are one of your early ancestors, a hunter who has suddenly come upon a ferocious animal. How you respond to the stress could determine whether you are the predator or the prey. Your adrenal glands pour out cortisol and adrenaline to mobilize sugar stored in your liver. As your blood sugar rises, your reflexes sharpen, your muscles feel a surge in power, and your ability to think soars sharply. Adrenaline causes the smooth muscle that lines your blood vessels to contract, and there is an increase in the chemicals that cause blood to clot. Both responses are designed to protect you if you are injured. At the same time, your pancreas senses the rise in blood sugar and releases some extra insulin. This rise in insulin serves two purposes: to push that glucose into your muscle cells for added energy, and to keep too much sugar from reaching your brain, which would be damaging. When you've dealt successfully with the situation, your chemicals and body responses return to normal. The crisis is over.

But what about chronic stress, the constant bothersome stimuli that nibble around the edges of your physical and psychological well being? The chemical reaction is the same as it is in acute stress, only at a lower level. And it doesn't end. If you're walking around angry all the time, or in pain, or seriously depressed or anxious, your cortisol and adrenaline levels are always elevated, even if not to the level of acute stress. Adrenaline is demanding a constant supply of glycogen to mobilize your stress responses in muscle and blood. And that adrenaline demand supports a constant flow of insulin to protect your brain and feed your muscles with sugar—except that if you're already insulin resistant, the sugar is stored instead as fat. And fat, as you know, contributes to insulin resistance. So chronic stress, whatever the cause, is the enemy of your efforts to combat insulin resistance.

Acute stress is unavoidable; we can't, by definition, know when emergency will confront us. Viewed in the short term, chronic stress may be unavoidable as well, but minimizing chronic stress is a valid long-term goal. Let's say that your daily commute to work is a chronic stressor. Traffic conditions are unpredictable; about once a week you find yourself in a traffic jam, flipping stations on the radio to keep yourself from boiling over, knowing you're going to be late to work, imagining all the things that will go undone or be done wrong if you're not there on time. While you're stuck in traffic is the perfect time to be thinking about how to minimize this particular stress in the future. Maybe a minor rearrangement of your morning routine might allow you to leave fifteen minutes earlier. Maybe the route you take to work needs rethinking. Maybe there is an alternative to driving by yourself every day—public transportation all or part of the way, or ride sharing.

The most stressful situations are those in which we feel we lack control. Merely deciding to look for ways to gain control is a stress-reducing action. On the other hand, sometimes relinquishing a measure of control is a stress reliever. If your chronic stress is partly because you feel overwhelmed by responsibility, perhaps a good first step toward stress relief would be to list all the things you are responsible for, and then for each item think about what would happen if you didn't take care of it, and, if it's absolutely necessary that someone do it, whom you might enlist to help. These are just a few suggestions about how you might approach chronic stress. The important point is that you need not just accept things as they are. You can approach the things that are causing you stress with the same will and intelligence that you use in the rest of your life. You can, and you must. Your health is too important to leave it to chance.

·15·
CHOOSING A LOW-CARBOHYDRATE EATING PLAN

PEOPLE WHO DECIDE to adopt the high-protein, low-carbohydrate way of eating face a bewildering assortment of diet books from which to choose. If the existence of so many competing low-carbohydrate plans leaves you stuck and uncertain where to start, this chapter will help you decide, based on your unique needs and preferences.

Of course, it's not necessary to read any of the books. You can, if you choose, decide how many grams of carbohydrates you will eat in a day, arm yourself with a book that gives the carbohydrate count for a variety of foods, assemble a collection of low-carbohydrate recipes (see the bibliography for books on carbohydrate counts and appendix 3 for sources of recipes), and get started. Having read this book, you already have the basic understanding of what you are going to do and why. Many people have succeeded in changing their way of eating and improving their health with less information than you have in your hands right now.

However, the various low-carbohydrate experts differ in some of their recommendations, and you will benefit from understanding these differences. In this chapter I review five of the current crop of books on low-carbohydrate eating. Some are best-sellers; some are not well known. Each is interesting and worthwhile in its own right. On the surface, any of the books listed in this chapter is suitable for losing weight, improving your blood chemistry, and reducing or reversing insulin resistance. On a deeper level, however, it is likely that some of these eating plans will work better for you than others. My aim in reviewing them is to give you an idea of the kinds of problems each addresses, the amount of discipline involved in each plan, and the relative ease of following each one so that you can decide where to start. It is common for people to try one plan and switch to another after weeks or months. I'll tell you about some people who have done that, and why.

Your choice of how and where to start making the lifestyle changes you need to make is especially important if there is a little voice lurking in your mind telling you that you'll fail in this effort, as you've failed before to change the way you eat. Your unique character and personality will determine which of these diets appeal to you and which seem less appropriate. For example, some of these diets require more advance planning, more record keeping, and more discipline than others. Some people like to plan and keep records; some do not. I'll tell you what it takes to adhere to each of these plans so that you can decide which best suits you.

Two mild warnings, should you decide to strike out on your own after reading this book. First, if you do not increase your intake of proteins and fats when you reduce your consumption of carbohydrates, not only will you not achieve the benefits of low-carbohydrate eating described in this book, but you will also find yourself tired, possibly depressed, and losing muscle mass. Experts disagree on how much protein you need and how little carbohydrate, but they agree that merely reducing carbohydrate intake is not the whole answer.

Second, some vitamins and minerals are more plentiful in fruits and vegetables than in proteins and fats. Vitamin C is probably the most important of these. It is important to your immune system and is necessary for the building of collagen, the protein that provides the framework for all of your body's tissues. Also, when you reduce carbohydrates, you will almost certainly get rid of a large quantity of excess water that you've been lugging around, but you will also eliminate sodium and potassium along with the water. Sodium is easy to replace; you pick up the salt shaker without giving it a thought when you are lacking sufficient sodium. The level of potassium required to maintain your blood pressure within normal limits, assure the proper passage of nerve signals, and keep your muscles functioning properly is a bit more tricky to maintain. Orange juice and bananas, two high-carbohydrate foods you will abandon when you enter the low-carbohydrate world, are the best sources of potassium.

The message here is that you will need either to consider vitamin and mineral supplements or to acquaint yourself with the best food sources of these and other micronutrients and be sure to eat them frequently. It will be a good idea to acquire a copy of *Earl Mindell's Vitamin Bible* and use it as a reference to point out the symptoms of any vitamin and mineral deficiencies and determine how you wish to supplement them. In other words, although the low-carbohydrate way of life is something you can adopt without additional information, you should be aware that deficiencies can develop, and that you may already have deficiencies in micronutrients on a conventional American diet that may not be eliminated when you switch to the low-carbohydrate way. You may decide to invest in supplements or you may not. The important thing is that you consider the possibility and inform yourself of your options.

You may wonder about the order in which the reviews appear. The answer is simple: I've arranged them in chronological order according to the year in which each book was first published. I did this so as not to imply that one is better than the others. Surely one may be more to your liking, based on your personal preferences. Here I've tried to give you the information you need to decide which one that may be.

DR. ATKINS' NEW DIET REVOLUTION

When *Dr. Atkins' Diet Revolution*, the predecessor to the current edition, first appeared in 1972, it stirred up a storm of controversy. While almost everyone else was advising people concerned about their weight to count calories, Dr. Robert C. Atkins, a cardiologist, came on the scene asserting that carbohydrates, not calories, were what really mattered. He may not have been the first to sound the alarm about Americans' enormous consumption of sugar, but because of his book's great success, his voice was the loudest at the time. So many people lost weight on the Atkins diet that its popularity led it to be branded a fad.

Within a few years, the low-fat diet had replaced the Atkins plan as the accepted way to lose weight. As Atkins points out in his *New Diet Revolution*, the 1992 revision of the 1972 book, sugar consumption increased even more when low-fat eating became popular. Controversy continues to surround Atkins, so much so that in 2000 the U.S. Department of Agriculture, which sponsors the carbohydrate-heavy food pyramid that Atkins and other low-carbohydrate advocates condemn as harmful to a great many people, announced that it will conduct a clinical trial comparing the Atkins diet with a famous and rigorous diet prescribed by Dean Ornish, M.D., another cardiologist. Ornish puts his patients on a vegetarian diet that allows practically no fat. The two diets could hardly be more different from each other. Results of the USDA experiment will probably be released in late 2001 or early 2002.

While Atkins addresses most of his book to people struggling to lose weight, the primary focus of his medical practice is heart disease. He was a pioneer in seeing the link between insulin resistance and obesity, diabetes, high blood pressure, and heart disease. Atkins lumps these conditions into a category he calls diet-related disorders (DRD) and asserts that most people who have DRD can be cured by following a low-carbohydrate regimen. To his credit, he does not claim that his dietary recommendations are the answer for everyone.

The Atkins diet consists of four stages. Stage 1 is called Induction. It usually lasts two weeks and is designed to force the body into ketosis. In the 1972 version of the diet, Atkins had his followers living on proteins and fats for the first week, then allowed them to add 5 grams of carbohydrates each week for a few weeks. In the current version, dieters eat no more than 20 grams of carbohydrates at first. This means three cups of most salad vegetables, or two cups of salad and two-thirds of a cup of non-starchy cooked vegetables. Meat, fish, poultry, shellfish, eggs, and cheese can be consumed in unlimited quantities. Atkins does not advocate restricting fats. Atkins says people's appetites automatically limit their intake of proteins and fats, and that most people will actually eat less fat on his diet than they did before they started.

First-time dieters may be astounded at the way weight seems to fall off their bodies in the first two weeks. Atkins acknowledges that much of this initial weight loss is the loss of water packed into cells by carbohydrates. Atkins's critics say this isn't true weight loss. But anyone who has ever lost ten pounds of excess water knows how much more comfortable it is not to be waterlogged. And as long as you stick to low-carbohydrate eating, that water doesn't come back, and before long you are losing fat as well.

Stage 2 Atkins calls Ongoing Weight Loss. It is a bit more liberal than Stage 1. In Stage 2 you add low-carbohydrate foods gradually, about 5 grams at a time and staying at the new level for a few weeks, to discover the level below which you can continue to lose weight. Atkins calls this the Critical Carbohydrate Level for Losing (CCLL). As long as your carbohydrate consumption stays below this level, you will lose weight. For about 40 percent of women, Atkins says, this level is only 30 grams daily. Others lose with more carbohydrates, or must continue to eat fewer. As you begin to approach your ideal weight in Stage 2, the weekly rate of loss slows down. Atkins says to expect it to take two or more months to shed the last ten pounds.

When you are within about five pounds of your goal weight, you enter Stage 3, the Pre-Maintenance level. Here you slow down your loss even more, increasing carbohydrate consumption until you are losing less than a pound a week. This is the time to learn what you can eat and still lose weight, even though slowly. It is a time of experimentation. You deviate from the low-carbohydrate diet by eating one or two higher-carbohydrate food items— a baked potato, a piece of fruit—in a week, watching your weight as you go. Ketosis will end during the Pre-Maintenance stage. When you get to your desired weight, you are in Maintenance mode, your way of eating forever. You know by this point how many carbohydrate grams you can eat without gaining weight.

If you have gone this far in the Atkins diet, you also know how to control your weight for the rest of your life: If you find yourself gaining, you go back on Induction until you lose the weight, then work your way through the steps back to Maintenance. For many people, the simple fact of learning that it is possible to control one's weight by adjusting carbohydrate intake is a life-changing discovery.

• *JOY: I started the Atkins diet on January 10, 2000. That was, as the saying goes, the first day of the rest of my life. To date [November 2000] I have lost 36 pounds, 17.75 inches, and gone from a tight size 24 to a loose size 20. What I have gained in return is indescribable, but I'll try.*

My cholesterol is 197. This is the first time in my adult life— I'm forty-one—that it has been under 230. I no longer have indigestion, flatulence, or the horrors of irritable bowel syndrome.

I have energy. I have confidence. I have fun. People at work are starting to compliment me regularly on my progress. I'm al-

ways amazed at how much nicer people are to me now. I still have quite a bit of weight to lose, but I'm optimistic it will happen. I am not in any hurry. One of my best friends at work lost sixty pounds in record time and has gained most of it back, almost as quickly. I don't want to follow that path. Once this weight is gone, I want it gone forever.

THE CARBOHYDRATE ADDICT'S DIET

By beginning their book with their own stories, Rachael F. Heller and Richard F. Heller, husband and wife doctors, demonstrate their familiarity with carbohydrate addiction. They provide a powerful antidote to the poison of guilt that afflicts carbohydrate addicts. Although they pay some attention to the psychological component of eating disorders, they show how a condition they call "glucose transport disorder" makes the craving for carbohydrates irresistible. Glucose transport disorder sounds quite like insulin resistance, and in fact after a while the Hellers stop referring to glucose transport disorder and focus on IR as the condition their diet is meant to combat. They do not, however, link IR to hypoglycemia, diabetes, or any of the other diseases and disorders I have associated with insulin resistance. There is no index entry for high blood pressure, and the only references to heart disease are in connection to low-fat dieting.

The essence of the Carbohydrate Addict's Diet is two high-fiber, very-low-carbohydrate, low-fat meals a day (called "Complementary Meals") and one "Reward Meal" in which you can eat as many carbohydrates as you care to, as long as you consume your Reward Meal in one sixty-minute sitting.

The authors provide a quiz to assess your level of carbohydrate addiction and point out that their eating plan is for addicts only. They claim a success rate of more than 80 percent for carbohydrate addicts who follow their instructions. The CAD defines three levels of addiction, from mild to severe. The eating plan is the same, however, for people at all three levels.

The theory behind their plan, the Hellers explain, is that the amount of insulin released when you start eating reflects the amount of carbohydrates eaten in earlier meals. They do not say how many prior meals enter into this calculation. The authors say a second insulin surge occurs 75 to 90 minutes later, this one determined by how much carbohydrate was eaten at the preceding meal. When insulin is finished doing its work and its level in the blood drops, the Hellers say, the decrease triggers a release of the brain chemical serotonin, which turns off appetite. Carbohydrate addiction occurs, they explain, when insulin levels fail to drop and there is no message from the brain that it's time to stop eating. Clustering almost all the day's carbohydrates in a one-hour period daily enables insulin levels to drop and appetite control to take hold.

The idea of the one-hour time limit on carbohydrate intake is that if you have finished eating at the time of the second insulin release, its amount will be low, while if you are still eating when the second surge occurs, it will be big enough to compensate for the release at the beginning of the meal, which presumably was low because of the two previous meals' carbohydrate restriction. They do not explain why there will not be a high insulin surge at breakfast on the morning following a dinner of unrestricted carbohydrates.

This eating plan stands in sharp contrast to the other low-carbohydrate diets reviewed in this book. Unlike the other low-carbohydrate plan authors, the Hellers see carbohydrates as the principal component of a healthy diet. Also different from the other low-carbohydrate plans is this book's approval of combining low-fat and low-carbohydrate dieting.

Although the book includes a bibliography, no footnotes in the text allow the reader to follow the authors' footsteps and see how they reached their conclusions concerning insulin releases and the relation between the postmeal drop in insulin levels and the release of serotonin. Various other authors have a different interpretation of this phenomenon, although I know of none that specifically disproves the Hellers' claims.

The diet consists of five distinct plans. Everyone begins on the Entry plan, consisting of two Complementary Meals, each containing no more than 4 grams of carbohydrate, and one Reward Meal. After the first two weeks dieters choose from among Plan A, B, C, and D each week, depending on how much weight they lost the week before and whether they want to lose or maintain their weight in the coming week. Plan D is the most strict; it allows only one Complementary Meal and one Reward Meal and requires that two cups of salad begin the meal. Plan A, the most liberal, allows two Complementary Meals, a Reward Meal, and a Complementary Snack. This is the only time that snacks are allowed at all.

The Hellers recommend losing no more than 1 percent of one's body weight in a week. For example, if you weigh 200 pounds, your weight loss in a week shouldn't exceed 2 pounds; at 150 pounds you shouldn't lose more than a pound and a half in a week. They advocate daily weighing, at the same time of day in the same kind of clothing (or none at all, as they recommend.) Daily weigh-ins should be recorded and averaged at the end of the week to find the week's average weight. This is very sound advice, for those who can stand to get on the scale every day, because the daily fluctuation in weight, even for a lean person, can be discouraging. For some, though, daily weighing may trigger self-defeating compulsive behavior, a fact that the Hellers do not address.

Complementary Meals must not include sugar or starch. The book's recipes make liberal use of artificial sweeteners. Some people with severe carbohydrate addiction have found that any sweet food can trigger cravings, even if the sweetener is noncaloric. While the book mentions the triggering capacity of monosodium glutamate (MSG), a chemical used in many foods and by many restaurants for flavor enhancement, it does not warn that aspartame can have the same effect.

The book provides a list of permitted foods for Complementary Meals, each of which should consist of 3 or 4 ounces of protein and two cups of salad or vegetables the book lists as permitted. Although there is no requirement to count carbohydrate grams, the book provides a list of the carbohydrate counts of common foods.

People who have tried the Carbohydrate Addict's Diet say it is not as easy as it sounds. A low-fat diet that allows only 3 or 4 ounces of protein at the first two meals of the day may leave you hungry. But while the Hellers recommend a low-fat diet, they do not require it. Most of the Complementary recipes offer the option of both low-fat and conventional fat ingredients. There is no prohibition of processed foods, chemical additives (other than the warning about MSG), or trans fats.

• BETH: *I started the Carbohydrate Addict's Diet at the end of November and loved it. I loved the Reward Meal and looked forward to it. The hour turned into a carb binge, and while I was hoping it would go away, it never did. I would stuff all the food I could get in my mouth within one hour of every day. I had lost weight after the first few months and was down a jean size but then I just stopped losing. My husband started talking about the Atkins diet, since someone he worked with was on it. I bought the book and decided to give it a try. So far so good. I think I'm much better off with little or no carbs than an hour full of them.*

• MAGGIE: *I think about what I'm going to have for dessert, but often I forget to eat it. I mostly plan fresh fruit. Fruit is my downfall. It's to me what chocolate is to [other people]. Last night I had strawberries, and tonight I'm going to have applesauce. This system works for me. I started it in October 1999 and am now [November 2000] down 54 pounds. I can wear a size 14 and shop in regular-size ladies' stores. And I do not feel deprived. I was on Atkins, and I avoided small children because if they were eating an apple I would have taken it from them! Now I don't even drool when I go through the produce section of the market.*

• CHARLOTTE: *I studied all of the plans and chose CAD. I only needed to lose 10 or 12 pounds. I ended up losing 17. I've never felt better physically, and I feel better looking than ever! I even have a new and final goal for next summer. There's no rush. I'm not even trying during the holidays.*

My Reward Meal usually consists of a slice or two of pizza, my favorite food, followed by one or more desserts, which include candy, cookies, cake, ice cream, etc. Am I controlling my carb addiction? You better believe it. Although I've never reached becoming obese, I've had to battle these constant cravings my entire adult life. I only start to gain when I'm cheating a lot. I didn't cheat once on my way to reaching goal.

And I don't think my cheating has anything to do with the Reward Meal, since many people on all programs fall off the wagon. I know I can jump back on the program and lose any excess pounds rather quickly (within the week).

PROTEIN POWER

If *Dr. Atkins' New Diet Revolution* and *The Zone* (a diet book by Dr. Barry Sears that is not included in this roundup because it advocates lower, but not low, carbohydrate intake) got married and had a baby, the baby would be Michael R. and Mary Dan Eades' *Protein Power*. This is the first book in the series of low-carbohydrate diet books to provide a thorough, nontechnical explanation of the relationship between a high-carbohydrate diet and many of the illnesses associated with hyperinsulinism. Like Atkins, the Eadeses approve of ketosis, although they don't make as much of a fuss over it as Atkins does. Like Sears, the Eadeses discuss eicosanoids and the importance of essential fatty acids. Like Atkins, the Eadeses base their recommendations on evidence gathered in the course of treating thousands of patients. Like Sears, the Eadeses argue for spreading the day's carbohydrate allotment equally over all three meals.

Protein Power is more specific in its recommended allocation of the macronutrients (proteins, carbohydrates, and fats) than Atkins, less specific than Sears. Its carbohydrate recommendation is slightly higher than Atkins, considerably lower than Sears. If there is anything to lessen the excellence of this book, it is the absence of footnotes and references to the Eadeses' source material. To make up for that lack, however, the authors invite readers to contact their publisher and ask for their bibliography. It is also available on their Web site (see appendix 3.)

Early on, the book provides a quick quiz, assessing the risk that you have or will develop insulin resistance. It goes on to describe a series of medical tests to have done before starting their eating plan. Each test is explained in detail, and numerical result ranges are given to help you understand the results. The Eadeses also provide a letter you can copy and show to your doctor if you are taking drugs to manage hypertension, fluid retention, high blood fats, or Type 2 diabetes. The letter explains that your need for these drugs will decrease while you follow the PP eating plan, and offers advice on how safely to taper off and eliminate these medications.

The book gives detailed directions for determining your lean body weight, the proportion of your body mass that is not composed of fat. True to its name, the Protein Power diet has you planning your meals around the proper number of grams of protein for your lean body weight. The Eadeses suggest that Americans tend to eat too little protein and are therefore in danger of losing muscle mass while they pile on fat from eating too many carbohydrates. They set no upper limit on protein intake, but insist on a minimum. Nor do they put a limit on fats, saying instead that fat shuts off appetite, and its intake therefore is self-limiting. The only other requirement, regardless of where you are in the plan, is to aim for 25 grams of fiber each day. In figuring the number of carbohydrate grams you eat, PP allows you to subtract grams of fiber from total grams of carbohydrate. There is also a calculator to help you determine your ideal body weight.

The diet proceeds in four steps: a two-phase Intervention

stage, Transition, and Maintenance. Total carbohydrate in Phase
I Intervention is 21–30 grams, distributed evenly throughout
the day. Because hunger is to be avoided, the Eadeses recommend keeping high-protein snacks always at hand. Two snacks
are allowed during the day, but the carbohydrate you eat in a
snack must be deducted from the next meal's allowance. You
move from Phase I to Phase II when you have reduced or eliminated any drugs you have been taking for high blood pressure,
blood sugar, or blood fats and kept your test results within normal range for at least four weeks. You are expected to stay at
Phase II Intervention (45–55 grams of carbohydrate per day)
until you have reached your desired proportion of lean and fat
body weight. People who have only a little weight to lose may
begin in Phase II at 55 carbohydrate grams per day.

The concept of lean and fat body weight is central to the Protein Power philosophy. The authors do not assume that every
reader is overweight. Rather than focus on losing weight, the
book talks about "recomposing" your body—changing the ratio
of fat to lean tissue. The Eadeses point out that your body weight
is made up of fat, lean muscle, and water, and that the objective
of overweight people should be to lose fat, not weight. The
Eadeses discourage frequent trips to the scale. Instead, they suggest using an article of clothing for reference to help you map
your progress. It should be something that you would like to fit
into. Periodically, you try it on and note your progress toward
getting it to button or zip. When you move from one phase of
the diet to the next, you recalculate your protein requirements
based on a new ratio of fat to lean body mass, which of course
does require getting weighed.

You enter the Transition phase of this eating plan with your
lean and fat body mass in proper balance, or when you are within
5 percent of your ideal body weight. Gradually, you increase
your carbohydrate intake, 5 to 10 grams at a time, until it is
equal to your protein allotment, much like Sears's *Zone*. Carbohydrate increases must be done gradually, the Eadeses warn, to

avoid insulin surges. A good rule is to stay at any new level for five to seven days before increasing again. Also like the Sears book, the Protein Power plan in the Maintenance phase calls for increasing carbohydrates above protein according to your level of physical activity. For physically active people, carbohydrate intake in Maintenance—that is, for the rest of your life—may be as much as 30 percent more than your protein intake.

The PP plan allows artificial sweeteners and says that diet sodas are fine in moderation. The authors place no limit on caffeine except in the case of those who are extremely sensitive to this stimulant. In them, caffeine may cause insulin surges and should be avoided. Wine and "light" beer are acceptable as long as their carbohydrate counts are included in the daily allotment, but distilled spirits raise insulin output and resistance and are to be avoided. The authors say that dry red wine may even increase cells' sensitivity to insulin—which is, after all, the main purpose of a low-carbohydrate diet.

The authors recognize that special occasions may cause plan adherents on maintenance to "slip," and advise planning for holiday feasts and accepting the consequences. The cure for a temporary lapse from grace is to go back to Intervention Phase I for three days, then Phase II for the rest of the week before returning to maintenance level.

One of the best features of this book is the restaurant dining guide. It suggests low-carbohydrate menu choices in various kinds of restaurants. The final section of *Protein Power* goes into detail on vitamin and mineral supplements, explaining why they are needed, how much to take, and even the best forms of various supplements. There are chapters on insulin-resistance-related diseases; one that makes a strong case for exercise, particularly weight training; and a discussion of eicosanoids and their role in inflammatory diseases.

• *CARLA: I've been on Protein Power for almost eleven months. I've lost over 117 pounds and have gone from 66 percent body fat to 34 percent body fat. I have rarely felt like I was on a diet except for a few longing glances at M&M's. If the carbs aren't eaten, the cravings go away. Also, I feel more active. I have no headaches. I stopped getting that sleepy feeling. I never am hungry.*

A month or so ago, my roommate went on CAD. I tried the program with her for the week before Thanksgiving. I neither lost nor gained any weight. I ate a lot of M&M's—and chips and desserts and bread. I went to sleep after every one of the meals, had amazing headaches, felt bloated and moody and generally crabby. I missed being in ketosis. I felt hungry. I would do the kitchen-prowl for food.

Basically, I eventually found that the diet wasn't worth it for me, and I went back onto Protein Power and went through a couple of days of carb cravings before I got back to the happy new me. For some people, CAD works great. But I am really an all-or-nothing dieter.

NEANDERTHIN

By the time he was thirty-four, Ray Audette was an insulin-dependent diabetic who had rheumatoid arthritis. Both diseases are related to malfunctions of the immune system. Audette set out to research autoimmune diseases and found that people whose food comes from nonagricultural sources (hunting and gathering, in other words) do not have problems with autoimmunity. He also learned that the occurrence of autoimmunity follows the path over which agriculture spread during the past 6,000 years. Audette decided to start eating the way the preagricultural people of the Stone Age did. Although he is silent on his current health status, he was apparently sufficiently gratified with his results to tell others what he has done.

Audette's theme is that eating foods made edible by technology is the underlying cause of numerous diseases of civilization. These diseases are not found among people who eat food as nature provides it. Audette extends the list of diseases that can be cured or at least improved by eating naturally to problems such as tooth decay, nearsightedness, chronic fatigue syndrome, acne, and emphysema. This is quite a stretch, and he does not provide testimonials from people who have solved these problems by eating like a caveman. But there is an active Internet community of people who stick to the so-called Paleodiet (see appendix 3), providing evidence that this diet is worth consideration by anyone with an autoimmunity problem.

Nature, in the context of the Paleolithic (Stone Age) diet, is defined as the absence of technology. This means that all foods you consume should be edible without any processing at all, including cooking. This is not to say that food may not be cooked—the book contains numerous recipes that require the use of an oven, Crock-Pot, or skillet. While Audette says that raw meat is most nourishing, he warns against eating commercially purchased meat without cooking it because of the danger of bacterial contamination. The author himself lives in Texas and hunts for his own food. He says that wild game is the best meat of all.

With this eating plan, no special foods are required. You can get everything you need from the supermarket, if you're not inclined to live as a hunter-gatherer yourself. Forbidden foods include grains, beans, squashes and gourds, potatoes, sugar and its substitutes, and dairy products. The question to ask yourself while shopping is this: Would this food be edible when found in its natural state, without applying technology (aside from heat)? The Paleolithic diet ultimately comes down to meats and fish, fruits, vegetables, nuts, seeds, and berries. Salt is not allowed. Sufficient sodium will come from meat, the author says.

Although this is not specifically a low-carbohydrate diet, it's almost impossible to overload on carbohydrates if you adhere to this plan, unless you emphasize the sweetest of fruits and ignore vegetables. People using this plan to lose weight or overcome in-sulin resistance should avoid fruits bred to be high in sugar—in other words, most commercially grown fruits. Caffeine is per-mitted in moderation. The book recommends green tea, which is low in caffeine and high in vitamins C and E.

Audette acknowledges that high-carbohydrate eaters will find the diet difficult at first, but says cravings will disappear after about a week. Those who experience the greatest problems with processed foods will also experience the most severe cravings, he says. Those who find the program most difficult to adapt to will also have the most to gain from it.

Hunger is not allowed. Those who follow this diet are en-couraged to eat as much and as often as they wish. Audette ad-vocates eating the widest possible variety of foods within the plan, in order to obtain the best combination of vitamins, min-erals, and other nutrients. The book overlooks the loss of nutri-ents that many observers have reported as resulting from transporting fruits and vegetables over long distances and some-times inadequate storage procedures.

A mainstay of the NeanderThin diet, and something that other low-carb dieters may want to consider, is jerked meat, or jerky (see appendix 3.) Homemade jerky should not be confused with the beef jerky available in grocery stores; the commercial version almost invariably contains some form of sugar. Pemmi-can, a high-energy food of Native American origin, is made of equal parts of powdered jerky and rendered beef fat. Audette says that 85 percent of the calories in pemmican come from fat, making it the closest equivalent in terms of nutritive value to mother's milk. He says it can keep for decades without refriger-ation and can sustain human life indefinitely without supplemen-tary vitamins or minerals.

The book includes ample tips for adhering to the diet at par-ties and in restaurants. Audette warns those who start the diet and then stray from its discipline that they are likely to experience a return of their former physical problems, quite possibly in a more severe form than they previously experienced.

That warning makes the NeanderThin approach seem like a last-ditch solution for people plagued with allergies or autoimmune disease. Adopting it is a serious commitment. If you are interested in this approach, you should first spend some time reading the archives of the discussion group that has grown up around it (see appendix 3.)

- MIKE: *This diet is difficult. Anything that puts me out of the mainstream is difficult. At dinner parties, socially, whatever, it's just hard. Lots of foods taste so good and add a lot to life's experience. We have learned to manufacture food that tastes really good but is bad for us, like a tailor-made mood-altering drug. I love Doritos nacho cheese, for instance. I wouldn't eat any, but sometimes it's in the house. . . .*

  Bottom line, it makes life a battle of stoic self-denial, unceasing wondering—should I have just a piece? just a chip?—and selective caving in with resultant guilt feelings. But the alternative is worse, I think.

- NED: *Frankly, the whole thing is, in the end, depressing. It is just tiresome to have to maintain such a strict rejectionist attitude toward food. As the years go by, it is in one sense "easier" to do this, but in another way it is increasingly tedious. This is why diets fail, of course. The mental energy consumed by this unceasing dietary vigilance takes a toll. When my vigilance flags, I gain weight.*

- MARK: *I have lost 111 pounds on the Paleo diet in one and a half years. I'm quite strict about my diet at home (except for about 3 ounces of cheese per week). I live alone and don't have non-Paleo foods in the house. When I go out socially I eat anything I want, with no guilt at all. So I don't have to cope with the social pressure. Limiting my non-Paleo food eating to restaurants and outside my house is one of the reasons I have been able to stay with this way of eating for so long. Another reason I stay on this diet is that when I go off it several meals in a row I feel sick emotionally, and eating seems to become my purpose in life.*

• DORIS: *At thirty-eight I was suddenly faced with a growing number of what doctors thought were symptoms indicating multiple sclerosis. I was experiencing extreme fatigue, cognitive, muscular, and neurological symptoms; my condition was rapidly deteriorating. I dove into the Paleolithic diet with a nothing-to-lose attitude, as my low-fat diet had failed me. To my amazement, all my symptoms began to disappear. Three years later I continue the practice of eating Paleo. I enjoy excellent health. Ridding my cupboards and refrigerator of all those processed foods was the best thing I ever did.*

When I first started eating Paleo and saw my health problems fading away, I was very encouraged. At that point I didn't care what it took, I was in for the long haul because I had already lived with failing health. I didn't like being sick or feeling like I was a burden to my family. So I was—and still am—very motivated. Literally, if I want to stay on my feet and feel well, I have to eat Paleo, so for me there really isn't a choice.

The diet has become easier over the years, partly because there are many people adapting, collecting, and sharing recipes. Don't get me wrong, there are times when I'd like to dive into an ice cream bucket headfirst. That's when I come up with some kind of yummy new Paleo-style dessert. I don't feel deprived of anything. I'm used to it, and if I want something, I figure out how to make a Paleo version of it.

Eating out can get a bit tricky, although I have only found one place in three years where I couldn't find anything on the menu to eat. It was a "health food" kind of place and served soy, tofu, and grain-filled foods.

LIFE WITHOUT BREAD

The updated English language version of Wolfgang Lutz's 1967 book *Leben ohne Brot*, this is more a clearly written book on the biochemistry of nutrition and disease than a diet book. The eating plan part of it is simple: Eat 72 grams of carbohydrate each day and as much other food as you wish. For Lutz and his American translator/coauthor Christian B. Allan, there are no other rules.

For more than forty years, Lutz has used low-carbohydrate nutrition to treat German and Austrian patients with a variety of ailments. He draws heavily on his own experience for his advice, yet the book is well documented with journal references in both English and German. Permitted foods are all fish, animal meats, eggs, cheeses, animal fats, salads, low-carbohydrate vegetables, and nuts. Alcohol in moderation is acceptable but must be included in the day's carbohydrate allowance. The only restricted foods are starchy carbohydrates—breads, pastas, cereals, grains, potatoes, pastries, bagels, sweet fruits, sweetened foods of any kind, and dried fruits—but even they are allowed within the day's 72-gram limit.

Lutz acknowledges that some people will gain weight on 72 grams of carbohydrates. However, those who are extremely thin may initially experience weight loss. These people, because they lack the energy reserves that body fat provides, have become accustomed to requiring an almost continuous supply of carbohydrates to meet their energy needs. After a few months, the thin person's metabolism will adjust and the production of growth hormone will increase. It may take a year or two, but eventually the consumption of fat and protein will result in a larger muscle mass, with the new weight deployed in all the right places. One of the book's illustrations is a set of before-and-after photographs of a gaunt man who returned to normal weight after eating Lutz's way for some time.

ginning with an explanation of the two kinds of nutrients the body cannot manufacture on its own—the essential amino acids and essential fatty acids, essential meaning they must come from outside the body—the book points out that there is no such thing as an essential component of carbohydrate. Human beings can live quite well without carbohydrates, but this book doesn't go that far in its recommendations. Lutz arrives at the 72-gram figure by calculating the glucose requirements of the brain and those organs that require glucose, and the time it takes to digest three daily meals. Eating 72 grams of carbohydrate will give you only as much as you can use during digestion itself. Anything more than that is converted into fat, Lutz says. He says that neither the very-low-carbohydrate recommendations of some diets (he doesn't mention Atkins, but that's who he means) nor the 40 percent carbohydrate requirement recommended for athletes (he doesn't mention Sears's *Zone*, but that's obviously what he's referring to) promotes optimal health.

However, the book never explains why, since there is no basic bodily need for carbohydrates, one should settle on 72 grams per day and not fewer. The body can use fats and proteins to supply its absolute glucose requirements. If it's not healthful to let this happen, nowhere does this book say so. Lutz sees no harm in ketosis, yet he prescribes a diet sufficiently high in carbohydrates to prevent it.

Whereas all of the other books reviewed here except Atkins's recommend minimizing or avoiding the intake of saturated (animal) fats, Lutz makes a strong case for including them in generous amounts. You have to eat large amounts of fat to overcome carbohydrate addiction, he says. Saturated fats are more chemically stable than unsaturated ones, and cell membranes made of saturated fats are less susceptible to oxidation and consequent cell damage. Warning of the danger in low-fat, low-carbohydrate diets, Lutz says that in some countries political prisoners are kept on a diet of nothing but lean meat as a way of getting rid of them. Within a few months they develop diarrhea and die due to lack of essential fatty acids.

Also like Atkins, Lutz sees nothing wrong with processed meats such as sausage and bacon. He says that small amounts of breading and carbohydrates in sauces need not be counted in the day's 72-gram allotment, but that larger amounts in items such as barbecue and sweet-and-sour sauces must be counted. The book is silent on the two controversies that swirl around the other low-carbohydrate books, artificial sweeteners and caffeine.

As an aid in counting carbohydrates, the book introduces a nineteenth-century concept known as the "bread unit," used at the time to help diabetics manage their blood sugars. A "bread unit" contains 12 usable grams of carbohydrates. In one place the book refers to a limit of five or six bread units. Everywhere else, six is the stated amount.

Lutz sees most modern diseases as the result of hormone imbalances caused by overconsumption of carbohydrates. In this list he includes diabetes, obesity, hyperthyroidism, heart disease, cancer, and "problematic sexual maturation." The book provides detailed explanations of how hormones act and how one hormone imbalance (that of insulin and glucagon) can trigger others. "Saturated animal fat and protein are the cure that stares us in the face," the authors write.

The book puts forth a theory of autoimmunity that is different from the lectin theory presented earlier in this book. It suggests that hormone imbalance may allow an autoimmune response to even a mild viral infection, causing Type 1 diabetes and multiple sclerosis. Whether the viral theory or the lectin theory is right—actually, both may be correct in different cases—Lutz's clinical experience demonstrates that minimizing carbohydrate intake is likely to reduce, if not eliminate, symptoms. Lutz is careful to point out that reversing symptoms is less likely as we grow older. Still, it's never too late to improve one's diet and hence one's health.

In writing about the constipation that often accompanies the early stages of low-carbohydrate eating, Lutz says to drink enough water to eliminate thirst but not more than that. Athletes and hikers, however, know that by the time you are thirsty, you are already dehydrated. And high-protein eaters are more prone to kidney stones if they do not keep themselves well hydrated.

Lutz warns people who are overweight and sedentary, advanced in age, or have diabetes, high blood pressure, or heart trouble to ease into the diet, beginning with nine bread units and working down to six over the course of a few months. Reducing carbohydrate intake is something like eliminating an addictive drug, he observes.

The book is more a detailed but highly readable explanation of metabolism and disease processes than a diet book. The chapter on energy metabolism is quite technical and may require more than one reading, but it's worth it. There are chapters on diabetes, heart disease, cancer, weight control, and gastrointestinal disorders, and even a section on nutrition for infants and children. There are tables showing the best sources for vitamins and minerals, debunking the myth that you must eat carbohydrates to obtain them. Several pages of tables are devoted to carbohydrate counts in terms of bread units.

Lutz tells people what to expect when they change their diet. Unfortunately, the book shows its 1960s origins where it recommends low doses of corticosteroids to overcome some relatively minor discomforts associated with immune system changes that result. This is an area that could have stood a fresh look in light of new knowledge of the effect of steroids on weight gain and problems such as yeast overgrowth.

This is probably not the book for serious carbohydrate addicts. Lutz says you can eat anything at all, including pastry, candy, or pasta, as long as you stay within the six-bread-unit limit. For people attracted to the Atkins way but wanting more detailed scientific information about the relationship between carbohydrate metabolism and disease, this book is highly recommended.

Which Plan Is Best for You?

The chart on the following page provides an easy reference to the main features of the five books reviewed in this chapter. The comparison is based on the following categories:

Min/Max. The minimum and maximum number of carbohydrate grams recommended.

Aspartame. Aspartame (NutraSweet, Equal) is the most popular artificial sweetener in the United States. Although most scientific studies have shown it to be safe, individual experience often indicates otherwise. Thus, its use in weight-loss diets is highly controversial. The chart indicates each expert's position on the use of aspartame.

Caffeine. Some experts recommend avoiding caffeine in a regimen designed to combat insulin resistance, some do not. This column indicates the position the author takes on this subject.

Alcohol. Indicates whether the diet allows alcoholic beverages. Where some are allowed but not others, those permitted are listed.

Deduct fiber. Similarly, experts disagree on whether to include the fiber content of carbohydrate foods in the total carbohydrate grams. This column indicates whether the diet allows you to deduct the fiber component when counting your carbohydrate intake.

Menus, Recipes. Indicates whether the book includes sample meal plans and recipes.

Low fat. Indicates whether the expert approves of a low-fat diet.

Snacks. Indicates whether meal plan provides for between-meal snacks.

Dairy. Indicates whether the diet allows milk and other dairy products.

Supplements. Indicates whether the author recommends supplementary vitamins and minerals.

Ketosis. Indicates whether the diet is likely to put you into the fat-burning state.

	Atkins	CAD	PP	Paleo	LWB
Min/Max	20/60+	n/a	21/55+	n/a	60/72
Aspartame	OK	OK	OK	No	n/a
Caffeine	OK	OK	OK	OK	n/a
Alcohol	Wine, spirits	OK	Wine, light beer	No	OK
Deduct fiber	No	No	Yes	n/a	Yes
Menus	Yes	Yes	Yes	Yes	No
Recipes	Yes	Yes	Yes	Yes	No
Low fat	No	Yes	No	No	No
Snacks	Yes	No	Yes	Yes	Yes
Dairy	OK	OK	OK	No	OK
Supplements	Yes	Yes	Yes	No	No
Ketosis	Yes	n/a	No	Yes	No

Key to Diet Plans: Atkins = *Dr. Atkins' New Diet Revolution;* CAD = *The Carbohydrate Addict's Diet;* PP = *Protein Power;* Paleo = *NeanderThin;* LWB = *Life without Bread.*

Choosing an eating plan in the face of such variety isn't easy. As you've seen, people often try more than one diet before deciding which suits them best. The following table is intended to make your choice easier by drawing on the experience of a few hundred low-carbohydrate followers. Pick the statement or statements that apply to you. The + symbol indicates relative goodness; the more plus signs, the better. Please don't choose your eating plan by adding up the plus signs. Rather, choose the characteristics that are most important to you, and let the individual ratings be your guide.

	Atkins	CAD	PP	Paleo	LWB
I am seriously addicted to carbohydrates.	+++	+	++	++	++
I am moderately/mildly addicted to carbohydrates.	++	++	+++	+	++
I have heart trouble and/or high blood pressure.	+++		++	++	++
I have diabetes.	++		++	+	++
I am seriously overweight.	+++	+	+++	++	++
I enjoy doing arithmetic and keeping records.			+++		
I don't like a lot of rules.	++				+++
I love dairy products; they don't bother me at all.	++	++	++		++
I won't stop eating processed foods.	++	++	++		++
A dinner without wine is like a day without sunshine.	++	+	+		++
I don't want to take supplements.		++		++	++
I have an autoimmune disease.	++		++	+++	++
I've dieted and failed many times.	++	+	++		++

You now have the information you need to begin, as Joy said in her comment about the Atkins diet, the first day of the rest of your life. You have, perhaps for the first time ever, the tools you need to control your weight and take charge of your health. You are about to step into a life of more energy and mental clarity than you imagined possible.

True, there will be a period of rearrangement and adjustment. Think of this as a challenge, a time of learning and excitement. You can do this. It's worth the effort. Nothing, absolutely nothing at all, is more important than the rest of your life.

·16·
MIRYAM'S SAMPLE MENUS AND RECIPES

THE QUESTION MOST commonly asked a person living the low-carbohydrate way is, What do you eat in a day? People accustomed to a high-carbohydrate diet find it hard to imagine feeling well-fed and enjoying your meals without breads, starches, and sweets. To help you imagine exactly that, here is what a day's food in the induction (ketogenic) phase of the Atkins diet (20 grams of carbohydrates or less) looks like. This is the lowest of the low-carb plans. Except for the Carbohydrate Addict's Diet, the others would include more carbohydrates at each meal. Carbohydrate counts for each item are given within square brackets [ ]. In giving carb counts I always round up, even if the fraction is less than one-half, and I always subtract fiber from the total carb count.

BREAKFAST
4–5 strips of bacon [0]

or

Cheese omelet [0.6 per egg, 1 oz. cheese = 0–1]

or

2 or more hard-boiled eggs

and

Tea (herbal, if possible) or decaffeinated coffee
[0; 1 tbsp. half and half or light cream = 0.4]

LUNCH
4–6 oz. can of fish (tuna, sardines, mackerel, etc.) [0–1]
Mayonnaise to moisten, splash of lemon juice [0–1]

or

4 oz. can of kippered herring snacks [0]
1 oz. cream cheese [1]

or

4–6 oz. of any kind of meat, poultry, cheese, or cooked
  eggs [0–1]

and

Green salad with dressing [greens 1, dressing 1–4]
Flavored sparkling water [0]

DINNER
Beef, pork, or chicken (example: Beefburger, steak, pork
  chop, baked chicken) [0]
2 cups of salad greens and 2 tbsp. dressing (*not* low-fat
  dressing) [greens 2, dressing 1–4]

or

1 cup of salad greens and dressing [1, 0.5–2] plus 1 cup
  buttered nonstarchy vegetable (example: broccoli or
  spinach) [vegetable 4, butter 0]
1 oz. macadamia nuts [4]

Total carbohydrates for the day: 9–20

If you try this for a day, you will see that hunger is not a problem. And this is a minimum-effort meal plan requiring no creativity and little cooking. Imagine what you can do when you get your hands on a collection of low-carbohydrate recipes.

LOW-CARBOHYDRATE RECIPES

Recipes are road maps, not commandments. Usually, the first time I try a recipe I do exactly what it says. The only adjustments I make at the outset are for sweetness and/or saltiness. From then on I adjust according to my own tastes and creativity. These recipes are the result of such adjustments.

Carbohydrate counts for some foods are given as <1 (less than 1 gram) for a given portion. But "less than one gram" may mean 0.9 grams, so if you ate six times the specified portion, you would be getting 5.4 grams of carbohydrate. In calculating carbohydrate contents of these foods, I've assumed that <1 means 0.9, and have figured accordingly. The actual count may be lower than the one given, but it won't be higher.

A word about desserts: If you are very insulin resistant and trying to lose weight, even low-carbohydrate sweets may stop your weight loss dead in its tracks. The main purpose of low-carbohydrate eating is to require as little insulin as possible. Some people have an insulin surge when they taste anything sweet, even if it contains no carbohydrates. If you make a habit of finishing your meals with dessert and find that you're not losing weight, this is probably why. If you can eat low-carbohydrate sweets without interfering with your weight-loss goal, consider yourself lucky, and enjoy.

CHOCOLATE PROTEIN BREAKFAST SHAKE
1 serving; 7 grams of carbohydrate.

Use whey or egg protein powder (from the health food or athlete's nutrition shelf). Buy it flavored or plain, but unsweetened (unless you like aspartame, in which case you should omit the stevia.) Each container of protein powder contains a scoop, which holds ⅓ cup. One scoop = 1.5 grams of carbohydrate. This recipe mixes equal parts of whey protein and unsweetened cocoa (1 scoop = 10.6 grams of carbohydrate.) The recipe calls for ½ scoop of each, for a total of 6 grams of carbohydrate and a delicious chocolate shake.

⅙ cup (½ scoop) protein powder
2 oz. heavy cream
14 oz. cold water, or cold water and ice to equal 14 oz.
10 drops liquid stevia (or artificial sweetener to taste)

Mix all ingredients in blender.

CRUSTLESS QUICHE
8 servings; 4 grams of carbohydrate per serving.

¼ lb. sliced bacon
½ lb. sliced Swiss cheese
2 cups steamed broccoli, spinach, or other low-carb vegetable
1¾ cups heavy cream
½ tsp. salt
¼ tsp. paprika
½ tsp. grated onion
Few grains of cayenne
3 eggs

Preheat oven to 325 °F.
Fry bacon until almost crisp, drain on paper towel.
Cut bacon into ½-inch pieces and arrange in bottom of an 8 × 11 × 2 nonstick baking pan, or lightly grease the pan if necessary.
Place the Swiss cheese slices on top of the bacon.
Then spread the steamed vegetables over the cheese.
In a saucepan over medium heat, warm the cream, but don't boil it.

Remove from heat.

Add salt, paprika, onion, and cayenne to the cream.

Then add eggs one at a time, beating after each one.

Pour into pan, trying not to disturb previous layers.

Bake until done, about 45 minutes. Center should jiggle when you shake the pan. It will get firm while it's cooling. Best served at room temperature.

LOW-CARB SPAGHETTI SAUCE
1 quart = 65 grams of carbohydrate.

- 28 oz. can tomato puree
- 4 oz. can mushroom stems and pieces (diced)
- ½ cup olive oil
- 1 tsp. onion flakes
- 1 tsp. Italian seasonings
- 1 tsp. garlic powder

Mix all ingredients in blender. Refrigerate for a day or so, to let the flavors blend. Use with Crustless Pizza, below, or on spaghetti squash.

EGG-CRUST PIZZA
Serves 2; 17 grams of carbohydrate each.

- ½ lb. grated Italian cheese mixture (Sargento brand Parmesan and Romano, for example)
- 4 ounces cream cheese
- 4 eggs
- ⅓ cup heavy cream
- ¼ cup grated parmesan cheese
- 1 cup Low-Carb spaghetti sauce (above)
- ½ lb Italian sausage

Preheat oven to 375 °F.

Beat together cream cheese and eggs until smooth. Add heavy cream and parmesan cheese. Grease 8" or 9" square baking pan with olive oil or cooking spray. Put 2 cups Italian cheeses in pan and pour mixture over the cheeses. Bake for 30 minutes.

Fry sausage, breaking it up into half-inch chunks. Combine with spaghetti sauce and spread over baked egg-cheese mixture. Top with remaining cheese. Bake until bubbly (about 15 minutes). Let stand a little while to set before serving.

REUBEN CASSEROLE
Serves 4; 7.5 grams per serving.

  1 medium onion, diced
  1 cup sour cream
  1 lb. sliced corned beef or pastrami
  ½ cup Thousand Island dressing (see below)
  1 jar or can (about 14 oz.) sauerkraut, drained well
  3 cups of grated Swiss cheese
  3 plum tomatoes, diced

Preheat oven to 350 °F. Lightly grease a 9 × 13 baking dish. Sauté the onion until transparent. Add sour cream and heat through, but don't boil. Remove onions and sour cream from heat. Arrange sliced meat on bottom of baking dish. Spread Thousand Island dressing over the meat, then spread the sauerkraut over the dressing. Add the onion–sour cream mixture. Sprinkle on the grated Swiss cheese. Arrange tomatoes over the cheese. Bake 30–40 minutes, until cheese melts. Let stand a few minutes before slicing and serving. This is even better chilled and reheated.

THOUSAND ISLAND DRESSING
About 3 grams.

  ½ cup mayonnaise
  2–3 tbsp. low-carb ketchup (see below)
  1–2 tbsp. pickle relish

Mix all ingredients thoroughly to a rich pink color.

LOW-CARB KETCHUP
Makes 12 oz.; 1.2 grams per ounce, or 2 tbsp.

6 oz. can tomato paste
3 oz. water
3 oz. white vinegar
½ tsp. onion powder
Salt to taste
3 tbsp. Splenda
Scant pinch of cloves or pumpkin pie spice

Mix all ingredients in blender. Store in refrigerator.

CHICKEN PAPRIKA
Serves 4; 11 grams per serving.

1 lb. onions, sliced thin
3 tbsp. olive oil
1 tbsp. butter
4 lbs. chicken pieces
2 cloves garlic, minced
3 tbsp. sweet Hungarian paprika
2 tsp. salt (or to taste)
4 tbsp. Dijon-style mustard
⅔ cup chicken stock (or water); more if needed

Sauté onions in olive oil and butter until tender and golden brown, stirring often. Add chicken pieces and garlic. Sauté, stirring until chicken has started to brown. Add paprika, salt, mustard, and some of the liquid. Cover and simmer until chicken is done (about ½ hour), adding liquid as needed.

SPICY ROAST CHICKEN

Number of servings depends on size of chicken. Carb count for spices is 10.4 grams; chicken is zero.

4 tsp. salt
2 tsp. paprika
1 tsp. cayenne pepper
1 tsp. onion powder
1 tsp. thyme
1 tsp. white pepper, ground
½ tsp. garlic powder
½ tsp. black pepper
1 large roasting chicken
1 large onion (needed just before roasting)

Combine the spices in a small bowl, mixing thoroughly. Remove giblets from chicken, clean the cavity, and pat dry with paper towel. Rub the spice mixture into the chicken, inside and out. Make sure it's evenly distributed and pressed deep into the skin. Place chicken in a large plastic bag, close tightly, and refrigerate overnight.

To roast: Preheat oven to 250 °F. Remove chicken from plastic bag and place in a roasting pan. Cut the onion into quarters, stuff it into the cavity. Roast, uncovered, for 5 hours. After the first hour, baste the chicken every half hour with pan juices. Let it rest for 10–20 minutes before carving.

As an alternative to the onion, pierce a lemon several times with a fork and put it into the cavity. The chicken will have a faint lemon flavor.

CRANBERRY SAUCE

The entire batch contains 12 grams of carbohydrate.

1 cup Splenda
1 cup water
12 oz. fresh cranberries

Dissolve Splenda in water. Bring to a boil. Add cranberries. Simmer 20 minutes. Cool and refrigerate.

CRUSTLESS CHEESE CAKE
Serves 12; 4 grams per serving.

5 8–oz. packages Philadelphia brand cream cheese
6 large eggs
12 oz. sour cream
1 tbsp. vanilla
Stevia to taste (batter should be slightly sweeter than you
    want it to be; it will lose some sweetness when you
    serve the cheese cake cold)

Preheat oven to 250 °F. Let the cream cheese soften at room temperature or warm it briefly in a microwave oven. Warm eggs by placing them in warm water. Warm an 8 × 11 × 2 glass pan. Butter the pan and set it aside. Combine all ingredients in a bowl and beat until smooth. Pour batter into the pan and bake 45–50 minutes. Remove while center of cake jiggles. It will solidify as it cools. Serve it directly from the baking pan with, if you like, a variety of syrups, such as Da Vinci sugarless syrups (the carbohydrate count does not include syrup).

ALMOND POUND CAKE
12 servings; 8 grams per serving.

1 cup butter
1 cup Splenda
5 whole eggs
2 cups finely ground almonds or almond flour
1 tsp. baking powder
1 tsp. lemon extract
1 tsp. vanilla extract

Preheat oven to 350°F. Cream butter and Splenda well. Add eggs, one at a time, beating after each. Mix almond flour (ground almonds) with baking powder and add to egg mixture a little at a time while beating. Add lemon and vanilla extracts. Pour into greased 9-inch cake pan and bake for 50–55 minutes. Cake will rise; it may crack in the center and then fall while cooling.

CHOCOLATE ALMOND POUND CAKE
12 servings; 9 grams of carbohydrate per serving.

½ cup butter, softened
4 oz. cream cheese, softened
1 cup Splenda
5 eggs
2 cups ground almonds
1 tsp. baking powder
1 tsp. vanilla extract
2 envelopes Nestlé's premelted baking chocolate
Preheat oven to 350 °F.

Cream butter, cream cheese, and Splenda. Add eggs, one at a time, beating after each. Mix ground almonds with baking powder; add to egg mixture a little at a time. Add vanilla and chocolate. Beat until smooth. Pour into 9-inch greased cake pan. Bake for 50–55 minutes.

APPENDIX 1
How to Read a Nutrition Facts Label

Nutrition Facts

Serving Size ½ cup (114g)
Servings Per Container 4

Amount Per Serving

Calories 90   Calories from Fat 30

	% Daily Value*
Total Fat 3g	**5%**
Saturated Fat 0g	**0%**
Cholesterol 0mg	**0%**
Sodium 300mg	**13%**
Total Carbohydrate 13g	**4%**
Dietary Fiber 3g	**12%**
Sugars 3g	
Protein 3g	

Vitamin A 80%	•	Vitamin C 60%
Calcium 4%	•	Iron 4%

* Percent Daily Values are based on a 2,000 calorie diet. Your daily values may be higher or lower depending on your calorie needs:

	Calories:	2,000	2,500
Total Fat	Less than	65g	80g
Sat Fat	Less than	20g	25g
Cholesterol	Less than	300mg	300mg
Sodium	Less than	2,400mg	2,400mg
Total Carbohydrate		300g	375g
Dietary Fiber		25g	30g

Calories per gram:
Fat 9 • Carbohydrate 4 • Protein 4

If you were counting calories and eating a low-fat diet, these numbers would be important. You're not, so you can ignore them.

This food has 13 grams of carbohydrate. Three grams are dietary fiber, so you can count the food as having 10 grams of carbohydrate, as long as you only eat the serving size (½ cup). If you have a cup of it, you will be eating 20 grams of carbohydrate.

The serving size does not mean that's how much you are supposed to eat. It tells you what amount of the food will provide the amount of protein, carbohydrate, and fat shown on the label.

If you must limit your salt intake, pay attention to sodium content as measured in mg.

Note that the label says you should eat 300 grams of carbohydrate if you're on a 2,000 calorie diet, 375 on a 2,500 calorie diet. This does not apply to people on a low-carbohydrate diet.

APPENDIX 2
Aids to Record Keeping

DAILY WEIGH-IN CHART

You can copy and use this chart to record your progress in losing weight, if it doesn't make you uncomfortable to do so. The only number that really matters is the average of all the times you've weighed yourself during the week. Add up all the days' weighings and divide by the number of days you've weighed yourself. You should expect your weight to fluctuate from day to day. If you are a woman, and it's around time for your monthly period, don't let a sudden weight gain upset you; it's water, and you'll lose it soon. Comparing this chart with your food diary may give you useful insights into what foods cause problems for you.

DAILY WEIGH-IN								
Week beginning (Date)	Mon.	Tues.	Wed.	Thurs.	Fri.	Sat.	Sun.	Week's Average

THE FOOD DIARY

Make copies of this page if you want to analyze the way you eat now, before making the changes needed to help you achieve your health goals. Once you have embarked on your new way of eating, there's no need to count calories, and whether you record proteins and fats depends on which of the diet plans you have chosen.

Please note: If you have an eating disorder or tend to be obsessive-compulsive about your eating, it may not be a good idea for you to go in for all this record keeping. The point of low-carbohydrate eating is to make you healthier and more comfortable, not to add to your stress. Please think about this before you begin keeping records, and give yourself permission to stop if it becomes a burden.

FOOD DIARY FOR (DATE) _____

Food	Quantity	Calories	Protein grams	Carb. grams	Fat grams

Day's summary

1. Total calories   _____
2. Total protein grams   _____ × 4 = Total protein calories _____
3. Total carb. grams   _____ × 4 = Total carb. calories   _____
4. Total fat grams   _____ × 9 = Total fat calories   _____
5. Protein calories   _____ / total calories × 100 = _____ % of
   day's calories from protein
6. Carb. calories   _____ / total calories × 100 = _____ % of
   day's calories from carb.
7. Fat calories   _____ / total calories × 100 = _____ % of
   day's calories from fat

If you set goals last week, you can compare them with this week's diary and set new goals. You may want to do this after you've looked at your weight chart for the week.

Goals for next week:

Total protein grams_____
Total carb. grams_____
Total fat grams   _____

APPENDIX 3

Resources

Finding foods and other products to facilitate a low-carbohy-drate way of eating need not be torture. The following five cate-gories of resources can help you locate everything you will need, including sites on the World Wide Web that offer all the support and information you could want, as well as information on e-mail lists, Internet newsgroups, and places to find recipes. Browse and enjoy.

PRODUCTS

Your local grocery store or supermarket has plenty of meat, fish, eggs, poultry, and cheese, and all the low-carb, leafy vegeta-bles you could hope for. Splenda, the nonartificial sugar substi-tute, is finding its way onto market shelves. Look for it next to the sugar. Stevia, another alternative sweetener, is sold in health food stores, which are otherwise not very useful for low-carbo-hydrate eaters because they generally cater to vegetarians.

Some condiments, such as ketchup and mayonnaise, may be loaded with sugars you don't want. Here you will find sources of low-carb alternatives. You can either browse the companies' Web sites or call them on the telephone and ask for a catalog.

Some of the recipes you will find, both in this book and in others, call for nut flours, which are hard to find in stores. You'll find sources for them here.

People who weigh more than 300 or 350 pounds are hard put to find a scale on which to track their progress when they change to low-carbohydrate eating. There's one in this list of products.

Carbsmart

Another excellent source of low-carb foods, including DaVinci low-carb syrups, sweetened with Splenda. Good, personalized service.

http://stores.yahoo.com/carbsmart/
877-279-7091

CarbWise Market

Another site where you can purchase low-carbohydrate foods and ingredients.

http://www.carbwise.com/disc.html
888-606-9280

Discount Natural Foods

Vitamins and minerals, stevia, and more. Excellent service; free shipping on orders over $20. Good prices.

http://www.vitaglo.com
888-418-8156

Expert Foods

Makers of Not/Starch, a fiber-based thickener for gravy, and other hard-to-find ingredients.

http://expertfoods@64.66.163.14/index.html
410-997-5155

High-weight scales

When you weigh more than 300 or 400 pounds, it's hard to track your weight as you start on your way down. The Fairbanks Portable Beam Scale has 1,000 lb. capacity. Item #19332, $449.99. Available at Northern Tool and Equipment Company

http://www.northern-online.com
800-221-0516

Low Carb Connoisseur

Browse a catalog of low-carbohydrate and sugar-free weight-loss products and culinary items for a variety of diets. You can find almond flour here.

http://www.low-carb.com
1-888-339-2477

Low-Carb Gourmet

Foods for low-carb living. Natural sweeteners, flavoring oils, and more.

http://www.lowcarbgourmet.com/store.html
800-569-1856

Low Carb Retreat

A good place to get started. Links to vendors of low-carb products, pages of information, recipes, a chat room for support and advice, recipes, mailing lists, and a set of frequently asked questions about the Atkins diet.

http://www.lowcarb.org/

Splenda

The manufacturer's Web site. Recipes (not necessarily low-carb, so beware), information for diabetics and health care professionals, articles, and more. You can find less expensive places to buy Splenda.

http://www.splenda.com

Total Discount Vitamins

Stevia, good prices on vitamins and mineral supplements.

http://www.totaldiscountvitamins.com/default.asp
800-283-2833

DIETS AND DIET BOOKS

These sites are controlled by the authors of the books reviewed in *Blood Sugar Blues*. When this was written, there was no Web site for *Life without Bread*.

Atkins Diet

> http://www.atkinscenter.com/

Carbohydrate Addicts Diet

> http://www.carbohydrateaddicts.com/

NeanderThin

> http://www.neanderthin.com

The Paleolithic Diet Page

A page of annotated links to sites for the Paleolithic Diet, also called a hunter/gatherer diet.

> http://www.panix.com/~paleodiet/

Protein Power

> http://www.eatprotein.com/

GENERAL INFORMATION WEB SITES

There are more than 500 Web sites related to the low-carbohydrate lifestyle. Here are just a few.

Balderon's Low Carb Recipe Collection

Create new dishes that are low in carbohydrates. Check out some menu options.

> http://www.photopics.com/lowcarb.html

Blood Sugar Blues on the Web

About insulin resistance, candidiasis, hypoglycemia, and fibromyalgia. (This book's Web site)

http://www.mwilliamson.com

Carbohydrate Contents of Prescription Drugs

Carbs are everywhere. You'll want to figure into your daily intake the carbohydrates in any prescription medicines you take regularly.

http://www.stanford.edu/group/ketodiet/ketomeds.html

Dietwatch

The nutrition advice isn't low-carb, but this site has a nutrition calculator you can use to track your macronutrient intake. You'll need to disregard the warnings that your carbohydrate intake is too low and your fat too high, but if what you want is a count of macronutrients in your food, this is a good place to go.

http://www.dietwatch.com/

The Glycemic Index

If you're interested in the glycemic index of foods, look here.

http://www.mendosa.com/gi.htm

How to Make Beef Jerky at Home

Beef jerky is a favorite, though expensive, snack for many low-carbers. Here's how to make it at home just like the pioneers did. This site also sells jerky.

http://www.jerkyusa.com/
800-322-0868

Insulin Resistance and Syndrome X Information
One of the earliest, and still one of the best. Reliable information and links to other sites.

http://commodore.perry.pps.pgh.pa.us/~odonnell/ir1.html

Jeff's Quick Carb Guide Page
On this page you will find carbohydrate counts for foods commonly eaten on low-carbohydrate diets. The listing of any particular food item is not an endorsement to eat it. You need to figure out for yourself what you can and cannot eat.

http://www.enteract.com/~jldavid/lowcarb/carbcount.html

Low-carb Recipe Exchange archives
These are the archives for an e-mail list called Low-carb Recipe Exchange. You can read and download recipes here. You can also join the mailing list and receive new recipes in your electronic mailbox.

http://www.egroups.com/group/low-carb-recipe-exchange/

Low-carb Vegetarian
Who says you can't be a vegetarian and eat a low-carbohydrate diet?

http://www.immuneweb.org/lowcarb/

Nutritional Counts at Fast Food Restaurants
Two independent sites that tell you what you're eating when you grab it and run.

http://www.dietriot.com/fff/rest.html
http://www.calorieking.com/cgi-bin/ck/fastfood.cgi

Nutrition Calculator
Another way of keeping track of the nutritional contents of what you eat.

http://homearts.com/helpers/calculators/caldocf1.htm

Recipes

There's no need to get bored with your food on a low-carbohydrate diet. Recipes are available in abundance online, and there are good low-carb cookbooks in every bookstore. You can start with the Web sites in the Diets and Diet Books section.

Tools for Counting Carbohydrates

You'll be surprised at how quickly you learn the carbohydrate counts of the foods you eat. But it's always a good idea to spot-check and be sure you're not letting extra carbs slip into your diet. If you stop losing and stay at one weight for a month or more, you may be on a normal plateau, or you may have let your guard down. These sites will help you keep track of your intake.

USDA Food Values Database

Don't be confused by the fact that this site lists "calories" as "energy" and with the more technically correct units of "Kcal" (kilocalories). The numbers are identical with the calories used on nutritional facts labels and in other nutritional databases. Type in the name of a food, and the system will give you a list of all the food items it has listed that contain that name. You then choose the size of the portion you want to know about. The result is a table showing the contents of the food: macronutrients, minerals, amino acids, and more. You can also download the USDA database at this site and use it in your own database management system.

> http://www.nal.usda.gov/fnic/cgi-bin/nut_search.pl

INTERNET MAILING LISTS AND ARCHIVES

Several e-mail lists are open to the public. You can read some messages on these Web sites, decide which you want to join, and join right on the spot. Or you can join by e-mail. Send a message to

> listserv@maelstrom.stjohns.edu

> with the message

> subscribe (list name) Your Name

In place of (list name) and without the parentheses, insert one of the list names below. They are the names after "archives/." Omit the letters "html" in your message. For example, to subscribe to Low Carb Anarchy, send a message that says

subscribe LC-A Your Name

You'll receive a welcome message that tells about etiquette on the list and how to manage your subscription.

Atkins Dieters Support Group

Another Atkins list. To subscribe, send a blank message to the address below.

Atkins_Support_List-subscribe@onelist.com

Dr. Atkins' New Diet Revolution

Support for Atkins diet devotees. You are expected to have read the book before you join.

http://maelstrom.stjohns.edu/archives/Atkins-new.html

Low Carb Anarchy

Freewheeling discussion, few rules, lots of support.

http://maelstrom.stjohns.edu/archives/LC-A.html

Low Carb Diabetes

http://maelstrom.stjohns.edu/archives/LC-DIABETES.html

Low Carb List

Not nearly as technical.

http://maelstrom.stjohns.edu/archives/
LOWCARB-LIST.html

Low Carb Technical Discussion

Provides ongoing information about low-carbohydrate diets for health professionals and those already well versed on the subject.

http://maelstrom.stjohns.edu/archives/lowcarb.html

INTERNET NEWS GROUPS

Internet newsgroups are much like mailing lists, except that you don't have to send a subscription message, and the information sent to newsgroups doesn't come to you as e-mail. Your internet service provider (ISP) chooses which newsgroups to provide from the 45,000 or more available. You may have to ask your ISP for a specific newsgroup. The ISP can also help you find newsgroups and tell you how to obtain the messages. Once you have downloaded the messages, you can read them and reply, just as with a mailing list. The difference is that you have to remember to download newsgroup messages, while e-mail messages come to you without any effort on your part, once you have subscribed.

alt.support.diet.low-carb

The main low-carb diet newsgroup. Lots of messages, not all of them pertinent. You learn quickly how to delete junk messages.

alt.support.diet.paleolithic

The Paleolithic diet newsgroup.

alt.support.hypoglyce\mia

Support for people with hypoglycemia.

http://www.grossweb.com/asdlc/

Frequently asked questions for the alt.support.diet.low-carb newsgroup.

Glossary

amino acids. Building blocks for protein; one class of micronutrients.

androgenic hormones. Also known as androgens, the male hormones—testosterone, androsterone, and DHEA. Smaller quantities occur in women as well.

antibody. A protective substance produced by the body's immune system in response to the presence of a foreign antigen.

antigen. A bit of protein that provokes an antibody response.

atherosclerosis. The condition in which fatty deposits build up inside blood vessels, narrowing the passage and eventually blocking the flow of blood to the heart. *Athero* comes from a Greek work meaning "porridge"; *sclerosis* is from another Greek word meaning "hardening." The term is often used as a synonym for *arteriosclerosis*, but it's actually a subset of that disease. Other things besides fatty buildup can cause arteriosclerosis.

autoantibody. An antibody that occurs in response to an autoantigen.

autoantigen. Material that is part of the body, but not recognized as such by the immune system, causing the production of autoantibodies.

autoimmunity. A condition that occurs when the immune system loses tolerance to its autoantibodies.

body mass index (BMI). A measure of the portion of total body weight that is made up of fat, as opposed to lean tissue.

candidiasis. Yeast infection or overgrowth, an excess of *Candida albicans*.

carbohydrates. Chains of sugar molecules found in breads and cereals, pasta, grains, starchy vegetables, fruits, most dairy products, and sweets.

cytokines. Immune system cells.

eicosanoids. Hormone-like substances that act within a cell, rather than between cells. These include prostaglandins, leukotrienes, and thromboxanes.

EFA. Essential fatty acid.

enzyme. A protein that can produce chemical changes in other substances without being changed itself.

essential fatty acid. A fatty acid that the body cannot make and that must be obtained from food.

estrogenic hormones. Also known as estrogens: the female hormones estriadol, estrone, and estriol. Smaller quantities occur in men as well.

free fatty acid (FFA). One of the by-products, along with glycerol, of the breakdown of fats in metabolism.

GERD. Gastroesophageal reflux disorder, heartburn.

glucagon. A hormone released by the alpha cells of the pancreas in response to too little glucose in the bloodstream.

glucose. A simple sugar that results from the breakdown of foods in the body.

glycerol. One of the products, with FFA, of the breakdown of fats in metabolism.

glycogen. Extra glucose stored in the liver and muscles.

gluconeogenesis. Literally, making new glucose; the process by which the liver turns stored glycogen back into glucose.

hormone. A chemical, released by a gland, that carries information or instructions to some part of the body.

hyperinsulinemia (*also hyperinsulinism*). Too much insulin in the bloodstream, evidence of insulin resistance in a person who is not diabetic and taking insulin.

hyperlipidemia. Too much fat in the blood, a risk factor for heart attack and stroke.

hypertension. High blood pressure. Blood pressure is reported as two numbers presented as a fraction, as 120/80 (said "one-twenty over eighty"). Blood pressure that is consistently higher than 130/85 (130/80 for diabetics) is considered to be hypertensive.

hypoglycemia. Low blood sugar; when it occurs after a meal, it is more properly called *reactive hypoglycemia.*

hypotension. Low blood pressure, usually considered to be any number lower than 90/60. While not as dangerous as hypertension, low blood pressure can cause falls and fainting, and in extreme circumstances can result in damage to the brain because of insufficient blood flow to nourish the brain's cells.

immune system. The body's way of protecting itself from invasion by germs and other foreign substances.

insulin. A hormone released by the beta cells of the pancreas in response to glucose in the bloodstream.

ketoacidosis. A dangerous complication of diabetes; not the same as *ketosis.*

ketones (also ketone bodies). A by-product of the breakdown of free fatty acids; a source of energy.

ketosis. The condition in which ketones provide energy in preference to glucose.

lectins. Minute plant proteins thought to cause some autoimmune diseases if they get into the bloodstream.

lipids. Fats.

lipolysis. The process by which stored fats are released into the bloodstream to provide energy.

macronutrient. Major component of all foods; a protein, carbohydrate, or fat.

metabolism. The transformation of food into energy and waste; all the chemical changes that take place in the body.

micronutrient. Components of macronutrients; vitamins, minerals, amino acids, and fatty acids.

normotensive. Having normal blood pressure.

NSAIDs. Nonsteroidal anti-inflammatory drugs.

osteopenia. Loss of bone. Leads to *osteoporosis,* or brittle bone disease.

polycystic ovarian syndrome (PCOS). A condition associated with insulin resistance, characterized by irregular menstrual periods and excessive hair growth in the male pattern, and often accompanied by obesity and infertility.

prostaglandin. One kind of eicosanoid.

protein. One of the macronutrients, protein provides energy and the amino acids necessary for tissue growth and repair; it is found in animal and plant foods.

Bibliography

Allan, Christian B., and Wolfgang Lutz, M.D. *Life without Bread*. Los Angeles: Keats Publishing, 2000.

Atkins, Robert C. *Dr. Atkins' New Diet Revolution*. New York: Avon Books, 1992.

Audette, Ray, and Troy Gilchrist. *NeanderThin*. New York: St. Martin's Press, 1999.

Bernstein, Richard K., M.D. *Dr. Bernstein's Diabetes Solution*. Boston: Little, Brown, 1997.

Burton, Gail. *The Candida Control Cookbook*. Lower Lake, Calif.: Aslan Publishing, 1993.

Cherniske, Stephen. *Caffeine Blues*. New York: Warner Books, 1998.

Gittleman, Ann Louise. *Get the Sugar Out*. New York: Three Rivers Press, 1996.

Coffee, Carole J. *Metabolism*. Madison, Conn.: Fence Creek Publishing, 1998.

Crawford, Michael, and David Marsh. *Nutrition and Evolution*. New Canaan, Conn.: Keats Publishing, 1995.

Eades, Michael R., and Mary Dan Eades. *Protein Power*. New York: Bantam Books, 1996.

Eades, Michael R., and Mary Dan Eades. *The Protein Power Life Plan*. New York: Warner Books, 2000.

Heller, Richard F., and Rachael F. Heller. *The Carbohydrate Addict's Diet*. New York: Penguin, 1991.

———. *Healthy for Life*. New York: Penguin, 1995.

McCullough, Fran. *The Low-Carb Cookbook*. New York: Hyperion, 1997.

McDonald, Lyle. *The Ketogenic Diet*. Kearney, Neb.: Morris Publishing, 1998.

Mindell, Earl. *Earl Mindell's Food as Medicine*. New York: Fireside, 1994.

Netzer, Corinne T. *The Complete Book of Food Counts*. New York: Dell, 1997.

Niewoehner, Catherine B. *Endocrine Pathophysiology*. Madison, Conn.: Fence Creek Publishing, 1998.

Reaven, Gerald M., and Ami Laws, eds. *Insulin Resistance: The Metabolic Syndrome X*. Totowa, N.J.: Humana Press, 1999.

Reaven, Gerald, M.D., Terry Kristen Strom, and Barry Fox. *Syndrome X: Overcoming the Silent Killer That Can Give You a Heart Attack*. New York: Simon & Schuster, 2000.

Rosenbluh, Edward S. *Elements of Behavioral Nutrition*. Louisville, Ky.: Behavioral Health Services, 1998.

Ruggerio, Roberta. *The Do's and Don'ts of Low Blood Sugar*. Sunrise, Fla.: Hypoglycemia Support Foundation, 1998.

Schwarzbein, Diana. *The Schwarzbein Principle*. Deerfield Beach, Fla.: Health Communications, 1999.

Sears, Barry, and William Lawren. *Enter the Zone*. New York: HarperCollins, 1995.

St. Amand, R. Paul, M.D. *What Your Doctor May Not Tell You About Fibromyalgia*. New York: Warner Books, 1999.

Williams, Roger J. *Biochemical Individuality*. New Canaan, Conn.: Keats Publishing, 1998.

Williamson, Miryam Ehrlich. *Fibromyalgia: A Comprehensive Approach*. New York: Walker & Co., 1996.

———. *The Fibromyalgia Relief Book*. New York: Walker & Co., 1998.

Index